U0275698

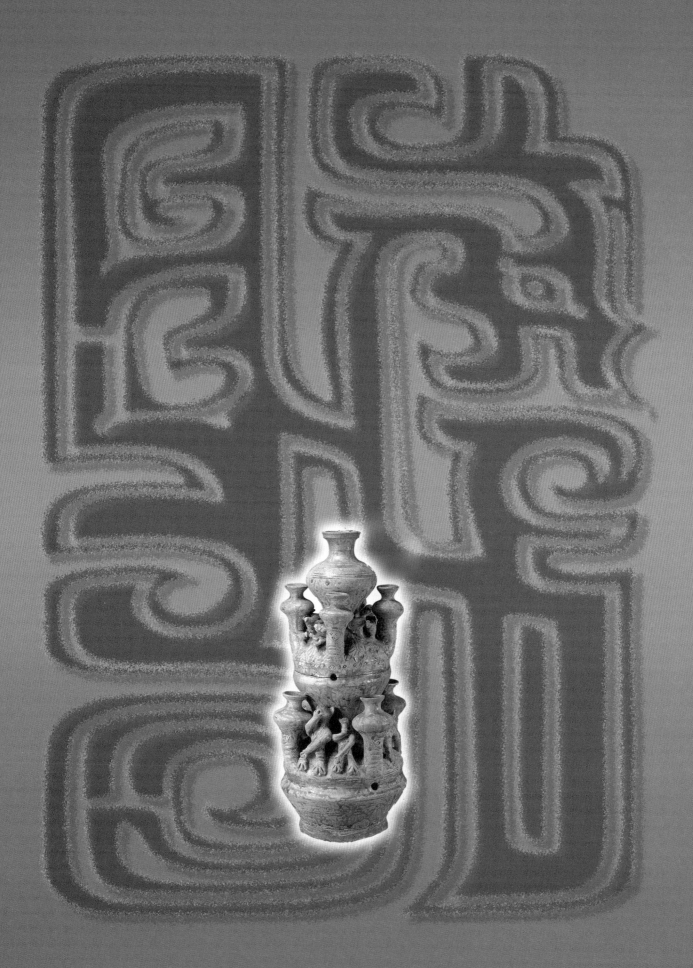

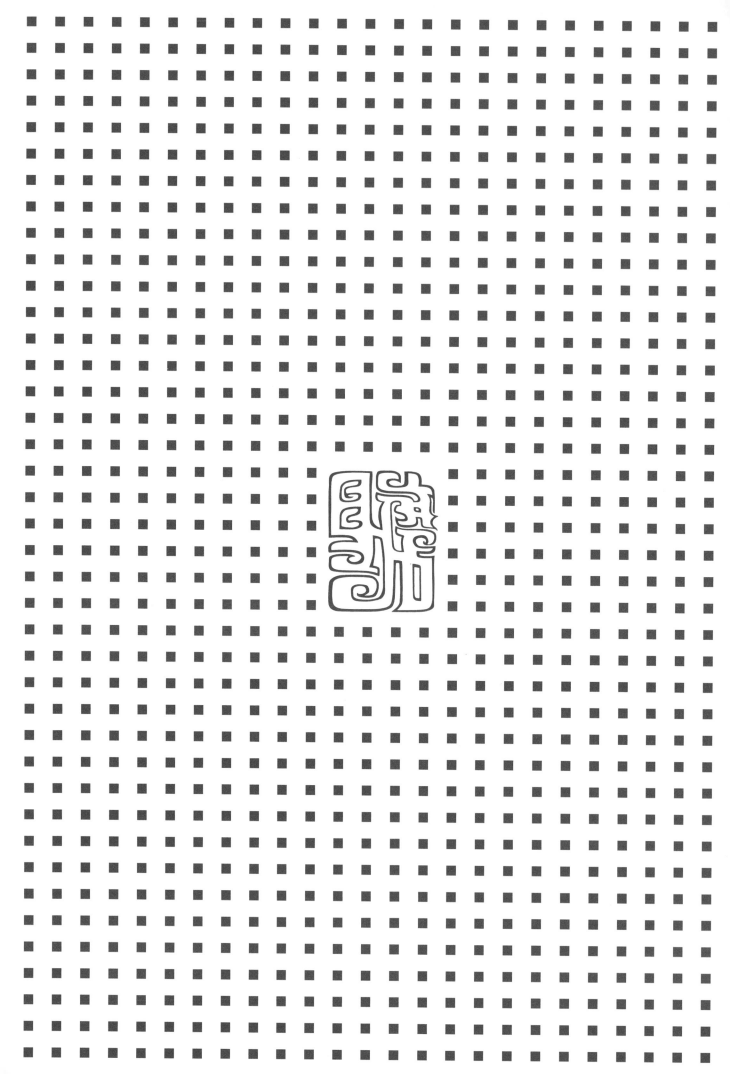

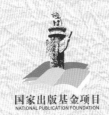

国家出版基金项目
NATIONAL PUBLICATION FOUNDATION

中华医药卫生

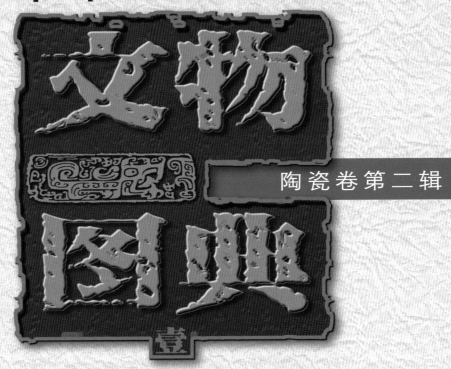

陶瓷卷第二辑

主　编　李经纬　梁　峻　刘学春
总主译　白永权
主　译　陈向京

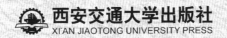

西安交通大学出版社
XI'AN JIAOTONG UNIVERSITY PRESS

图书在版编目（CIP）数据

中华医药卫生文物图典 . 1. 陶瓷卷 . 第 2 辑 . / 李经纬，

梁峻，刘学春主编 .— 西安：西安交通大学出版社，2016.12

ISBN 978-7-5605-7029-7

Ⅰ . ①中… Ⅱ . ①李… ②梁…③刘… Ⅲ . ①中国医药学 –

古代陶瓷 – 中国 – 图录 Ⅳ . ① R-092 ② K870.2

中国版本图书馆 CIP 数据核字（2015）第 013564 号

书　　名	中华医药卫生文物图典（一）陶瓷卷第二辑
主　　编	李经纬　梁　峻　刘学春
责任编辑	赵文娟

出版发行	西安交通大学出版社
	（西安市兴庆南路 10 号　邮政编码 710049）
网　　址	http://www.xjtupress.com
电　　话	（029）82668805 82668502（医学分社）
	（029）82668315（总编办）
传　　真	（029）82668280
印　　刷	中煤地西安地图制印有限公司

开　　本	889mm×1194mm　1/16　印张 31.5　字数 511 千字
版次印次	2017 年 12 月第 1 版　2017 年 12 月第 1 次印刷
书　　号	ISBN 978-7-5605-7029-7
定　　价	980.00 元

读者购书、书店添货、如发现印装质量问题，请通过以下方式联系、调换。

订购热线：（029）82665248　（029）82665249

投稿热线：（029）82668805　（029）82668502

读者信箱：medpress@126.com

版权所有　侵权必究

铭记感受历史

自信自重自强

中华医药卫生文物图典问世 书贺

陈可冀 谨题

二〇一七年春月

陈可冀　中国科学院院士、国医大师

精修醫藥衛生文物

圖典功著當代

深究岐黃學術思想

淵源惠澤千秋

中華醫藥衛生文物圖典出版誌慶

丁酉孟秋 孫光榮 敬題於北京

孫光荣　国医大师

中華醫藥衛生文物圖典出版

彰顯中醫藥
文化精神

體現中醫藥
歷史價值

歲次丁酉夏 王琦

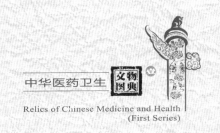

中华医药卫生

Relics of Chinese Medicine and Health
(First Series)

中华医药卫生文物图典（一）
丛书编撰委员会

主　编　李经纬　梁　峻　刘学春

副主编　廖　果　吴鸿洲　康兴军　和中浚　刘小斌　杨金生

　　　　郑怀林　徐江雁　白建疆　黄　煌

编　委　李洪晓　梁永宣　王强虎　董树平　马　健　王　霞

　　　　张雅宗　朱德明　包哈申　张建青　郑　蓉　庄乾竹

　　　　李宏红　刘哲峰　王宏才　陈润东

总主译　白永权

主　译　陈向京　聂文信　范晓晖　温　睿　赵永生　杜彦龙

　　　　吉　乐　李小棉　郭　梦　陈　曦

副主译（按姓氏音序排列）

　　　　董艳云　姜雨孜　李建西　刘　慧　马　健　任宝磊

　　　　任　萌　任　莹　王　颇　习通源　谢皖吉　徐素云

　　　　许崇钰　许　梅　詹菊红　赵　菲　邹郝晶

译　者（按姓氏音序排列）

迟征宇　邓　甜　付一豪　高　琛　高　媛　郭　宁

韩　蕾　何宗昌　胡勇强　黄　鋆　蒋新蕾　康晓薇

李静波　刘雅恬　刘妍萌　鲁显生　马　月　牛笑语

唐云鹏　唐臻娜　田　多　铁红玲　佟健一　王　晨

王　丹　王　栋　王　丽　王　媛　王慧敏　王梦杰

王仙先　吴耀均　席　慧　肖国强　许子洋　闫红贤

杨姣姣　姚　晔　张　阳　张　鋆　张继飞　张梦原

张晓谦　赵　欣　赵亚力　郑　青　郑艳华　朱江嵩

朱瑛培

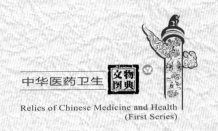

中华医药卫生文物图典

Relics of Chinese Medicine and Health
(First Series)

本册编撰委员会

主　编　李经纬　梁　峻　刘学春

副主编　廖　果　吴鸿洲　康兴军　和中浚　刘小斌　杨金生

　　　　郑怀林　徐江雁　白建疆　黄　煌

编　委　李洪晓　梁永宣　王强虎　董树平　马　健　王　霞

　　　　张雅宗　朱德明　包哈申　张建青　郑　蓉　庄乾竹

　　　　李宏红　刘哲峰　王宏才　陈润东

总主译　白永权

主　译　陈向京

副主译　邹郝晶

译　者　董艳云　许　梅　王梦杰　高　媛　王　丽　张晓谦

　　　　许子洋　王　晨　郑艳秋　刘妍萌

丛书策划委员会

丛书总策划　王强虎　王宏才　李　晶　秦金霞

统 筹 人 员　王强虎

丛 书 外 审　王宏才

编辑委员会　王强虎　李　晶　赵文娟　张沛烨　秦金霞　王　磊
　　　　　　　郭泉泉　郅梦杰　田　滢　张静静

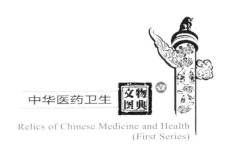

中华医药卫生 文物图典

Relics of Chinese Medicine and Health
(First Series)

序 言

　　探索天、地、人运动变化规律以及"气化物生"过程的相互关系，是人类永恒的课题。宇宙不可逆，地球不可逆，人生不可逆业已成为共识。天地造化形成自然，人类活动构成文化。文物既是文化的载体，又是物化的历史，还是文明的见证。

　　追求健康长寿是人类共同的夙愿。中华民族之所以繁衍昌盛，健康文化起了巨大的推动作用。由于古人谋求生存发展、应对环境变化产生的智慧，大多反映在以医药卫生为核心的健康文化之中，所以，习总书记说："中医药学是中国古代科学的瑰宝，也是打开中华文明宝库的钥匙"。

　　秉持文化大发展、大繁荣理念，中国中医科学院李经纬、梁峻等为负责人的科研团队在完成科技部"国家重点医药卫生文物收集调研和保护"课题获 2005 年度中华中医药学会科技二等奖基础上，又资鉴"夏商周断代工程""中华文明探源工程"等相关考古成果，用有重要价值的新出土文物置换原拍摄质量较差的文物，适当补充民族医药文物，共精选收载 5000 余件。经西安交通大学出版社申报，《中华医药卫生文物图典（一）》（以下简称《图典》）于 2013 年获得了国家出版基金的资助，并经专业翻译团队翻译，使《图典》得以面世。

　　文物承载的信息多元丰富，发掘解读其中蕴藏的智慧并非易事。 医药卫生文物更具有特殊性，除文物的一般属性外，还承载着传统医学发展史迹与促进健康的信息。运用历史唯物主义观察发掘文物信息，善于从生活文物中领悟卫生信息，才能准确解读其功能，也才能诠释其在民生健康中的历史作用，收到以古鉴今之效果。"历史是现实的根源"，任何一个民族都不能割断历史，史料都包含在文化中。"文化是民族的血脉，是人民的精神家园"，文化繁荣才能实现中华民族的伟大复兴。值本《图典》付梓之际，用"梳理文化之脉，必获健康之果"作为序言并和作者、读者共勉！

中央文史研究馆馆员
中国工程院院士　　王永炎
丁酉年仲夏

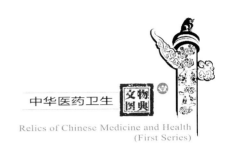

中华医药卫生文物图典

Relics of Chinese Medicine and Health
(First Series)

前　言

　　文化是相对自然的概念，是考古界常用词汇。文物是文化的重要组成部分，既是文明的物证，又是物化的历史。狭义医药卫生文物是疾病防治模式语境下的解读，而广义医药卫生文物则是躯体、心态、环境适应三维健康模式下的诠释。中华民族是 56 个民族组成的多元一体大家庭，中华医药卫生文物当然包括各民族的健康文化遗存。

　　天地造化如造山、板块漂移、气候变迁、生物起源进化等形成自然。气化物生莫贵于人，即整个生物进化的最高成果是人类自身。广义而言，人类生存思维留下的痕迹即物质财富和精神财富总和构成文化，其一般的物化形式是视觉感知的文物、文献、胜迹等。其中质变标志明晰的文化如文字、文物、城市、礼仪等可称作文明。从唯物史观视角观察，狭义文化即精神财富，尤其体现人类精、气、神状态的事项，其本质也具有特殊物质属性，如量子也具有波粒二相性，这种粒子也是物质，无非运动方式特殊而已。现代所谓可重复验证的"科学"，事实上也是从文化中分离出来的事项，因此也是一种特殊文化形式。追求健康长寿是人类共同的夙愿。中华民族之所以繁衍昌盛，是因为健康文化异彩纷呈。中华优秀传统医药文化之所以博大精深，是因为其原创思维博大、格物致知精深，所以，习总书记说："中医药学是中国古代科学的瑰宝，也是打开中华文明宝库的钥匙"。

文化既反映时代、地域、民族分布、生产资料来源、技术水平等信息，又反映人类认知水平和生存智慧。发掘解读文物、文献中蕴藏的健康知识和灵动智慧，首先是从事健康工作者的责任和义务。《易经》设有"观"卦，人类作为观察者，不仅要积极收藏展陈文物，而且要善于捕捉文物倾诉的信息，汲取养分，启迪思维，收到古为今用之效果。墨子三表法，首先一表即"本之于古者圣王之事"，也是强调古代史实的重要性。"历史是现实的根源"，现实是未来的基础。任何一个国家、地区、民族都不能割断历史、忽略基础，这个基础就是文化。"文化是民族的血脉，是人民的精神家园"。文化繁荣才能驱动各项事业发展，才能实现中华民族的伟大复兴。

人类从类人猿分化出来。"禄丰古猿禄丰种"是云南禄丰发现的类人猿化石，距今七八百万年。距今 200 万年前人类进入旧石器时代，直立行走，打制石器产生工具意识，管理火种，是所谓"燧人氏"时代。中国留存有更新世早、中期的元谋、蓝田、北京人等遗址。距今 10 万—5 万年前，人类进入旧石器时代中期，即早期智人阶段，脑容量增加，和欧洲、非洲人种相比，原始蒙古人种颧骨前突等，是所谓"伏羲氏"时代。中国发现的马坝、长阳、丁村人等较典型。距今 5 万—1 万年前，人类进入旧石器时代晚期，即晚期智人阶段，细石器、骨角器等遍布全国，山顶洞、柳江、资阳人等较典型。

中石器时代距今约 1 万年，是旧石器时代向新石器时代的短暂过渡期，弓箭发明，狗被驯化。河南灵井、陕西沙苑遗址等作为代表。距今 1 万—公元前 2600 年前后，人类进入新石器时代，磨光石器、烧制陶器，出现农业村落并饲养家畜，是所谓"神农氏"时代。公元前 7000 年以来，在甲、骨、陶、石等载体上出现契刻符号、七音阶骨笛乐器等，反映出人文气息趋浓。公元前 6000—公元前 3500 年的老官台、裴李岗、河姆渡、马家浜、仰韶等文化遗址，彰显出先民围绕生存健康问题所做的各种努力。

公元前 4800 年以来，以关中、晋南、豫西为中心形成的仰韶文化，是中原史前文化的重要标志。以半坡、庙底沟类型为典型，自公元前 3500 年走向繁荣，属于锄耕粟黍稻兼营渔猎饲养猪鸡经济方式，彩陶尤其发达。公元前 4400—公元前 3300 年，长江中游的大溪文化，薄胎彩陶和白陶发达。公元前 4300—公元前 2500 年山东丰岛的大汶口文化，红陶为主。公元前 3500 年前后，辽东的红山文化原始宗教发展。公元前 3300 年以来，长江下游由河姆渡、马家浜文化衍续的良渚文化和陇西的马家窑文化、江淮间的薛家岗文化时趋发达。

公元前 2600—公元前 2000 年，黄河中下游龙山文化群形成，冶铸铜器，制作玉器，土坯、石灰、夯筑技术开始应用。公元前 2697 年，轩辕战败炎帝（有说其后裔）、蚩尤而为黄帝纪元元年。黄帝西巡访贤，"至岐见岐伯，引载而归，访于治道"。其引归地"溱洧襟带于前，梅泰环拱于后"，即今河南新密市古城寨。岐黄答问，构建《黄帝内经》健康知识体系，中华文明从关注民生健康起步。颛顼改革宗教，神职人员出现；帝喾修身节用，帝尧和合百国，舜同律度量衡，大禹疏导治水，中华民族不断繁衍昌盛。

公元前 2070 年，禹之子启以豫西晋南为中心建立夏王朝，二里头青铜文化为其特征，半地穴、窑洞、地面建筑并存。饮食卫生器具、酒器增多。朱砂安神作用在宫殿应用。公元前 1600 年，商灭夏。偃师商城设有铸铜作坊。公元前 1300 年，盘庚迁殷，使用甲骨文。武丁时期青铜浑铸、分铸并存。公元前 1056 年，相传周"文王被殷纣拘于羑里，演《周易》，成六十四卦"。公元前 1046 年，武王克商建周，定都镐京。青铜器始铸长篇铭文，周原发掘出微型甲骨文字。公元前 770 年，平王东迁。虢国铸铜柄铁剑。公元前 753 年，秦国设置史官。公元前 707 年出现蝗灾、公元前 613 年出现"哈雷彗星"，均被孔子载入《春秋》。公元前 221 年，秦始皇统一中国，多元一体民族大家庭形成，中华医药卫生文物异彩纷呈。

中国是治史大国，历来重视发展文化博物事业，1955 年成立卫生部中医研究院时就设置医史研究室，1982 年中国医史文献研究所成立时复建中国医史博物馆研究收藏展陈文物。2000—2003 年，经王永炎院士、姚乃礼院长等呼吁，科技部批准立项，由李经纬、梁峻为负责人的团队完成"国家重点医药卫生文物收集调研和保护"项目任务，受到科技部项目验收组专家的高度评价，获中华中医药学会科技进步二等奖。2013 年，在国家出版基金资助下，课题组对部分文物重新拍摄或必要置换、充实民族医药文物后，由西安交通大学出版社编辑、组聘国内一流翻译团队英译说明文字付梓，受到国家中医药博物馆筹备工作领导小组和办公室的高度重视。

"物以类聚"，《图典》主要依据文物质地、种类分为 9 卷，计有陶瓷，金属，纸质，竹木，玉石、织品及标本，壁画石刻及遗址，

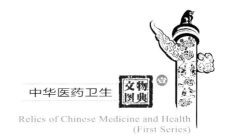

中华医药卫生 文物图典

Relics of Chinese Medicine and Health
(First Series)

Contents

Chapter Three   Three Kingdoms Period

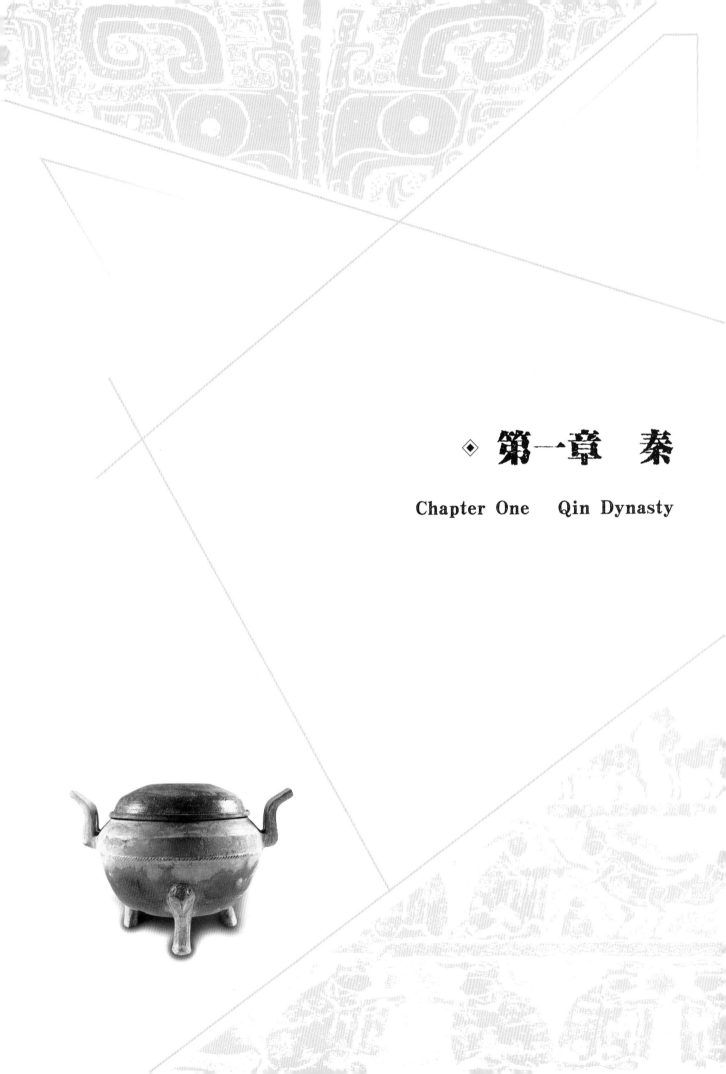

◆ 第一章 秦

Chapter One   Qin Dynasty

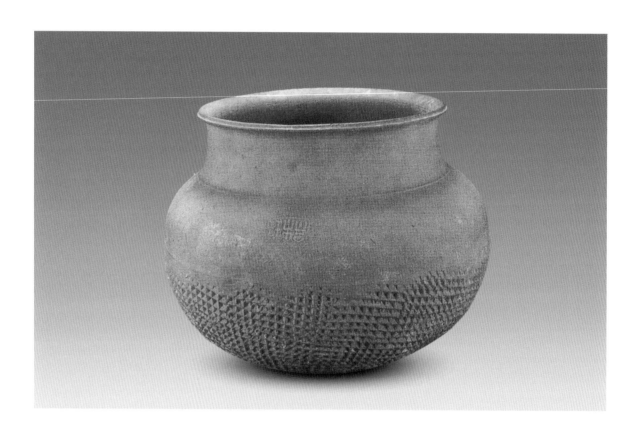

红陶釜

秦

夹砂红陶质

口径 17 厘米，通高 17.5 厘米

Red Pottery "Fu"(Kettle)

Qin Dynasty

Red Sandy Pottery

Mouth Diameter 17 cm/ Height 17.5 cm

肩部有凹的方胜纹，完整精美。炊具。1981
年于陕西咸阳采集。

陕西医史博物馆藏

The shoulder of this kettle is decorated with concave rhombus designs. This exquisitely-designed kettle remains intact. It was used as a cooker and was unearthed from Xianyang City, Shaanxi Province.

Preserved in Shaanxi Museum of Medical History

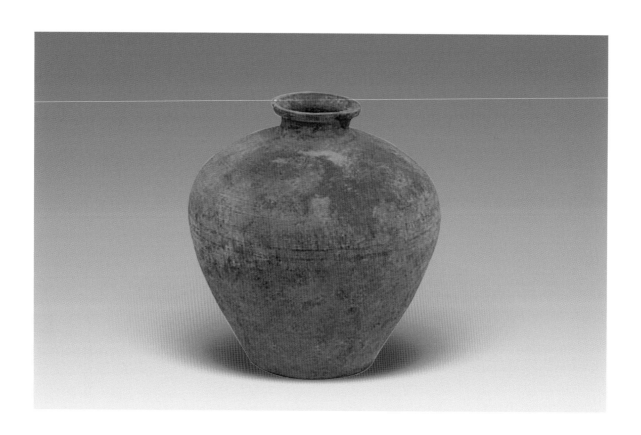

药酒坛

秦

陶瓷质

最大直径 60 厘米，高 60 厘米

Medical Wine Jar

Qin Dynasty

Pottery and Porcelain

Maximal Diameter 60 cm/ Height 60 cm

侈口，折沿，短颈，溜肩，鼓腹，平底，圈足。肩部刻有铭文，其大意是"大富贵，保健康"。用于盛装药酒。

北京御生堂中医药博物馆藏

The jar has a widely flared mouth, a folded rim, a bulged belly, a flat bottom, a ring foot, a short neck and a narrow and inclined shoulder. The shoulder is carved with the inscription meaning prosperous and healthy. It was used for storing the medical wine.

Preserved in Chinese Medicine Museum of Beijing Yu Sheng Tang Drugstore

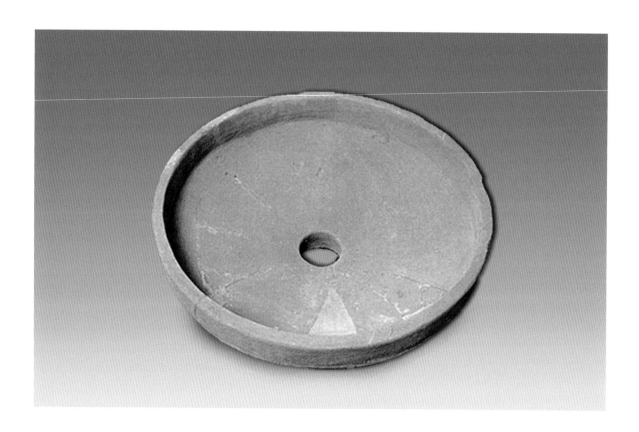

渗井□

秦

陶质

大口径 94 厘米，小口径 13 厘米，高 33 厘米

Filter Well □

Qin Dynasty

Pottery

Big Mouth Diameter 94 cm/ Small Mouth Diameter 13 cm/ Height 33 cm

直口，斜底漏斗状，是宫内排污设施，其下接

有虹吸的排水管。陕西咸阳秦宫一号遗址出土。

陕西医史博物馆藏

With a straight mouth and a slant funnel-shaped
bottom, this utensil is connected to a siphon
tube on the bottom. It served as sewage disposal
facility, and was excavated from No.1 Site of Qin
Palace in Xianyang City, Shaanxi Province.
Preserved in Shaanxi Museum of Medical History

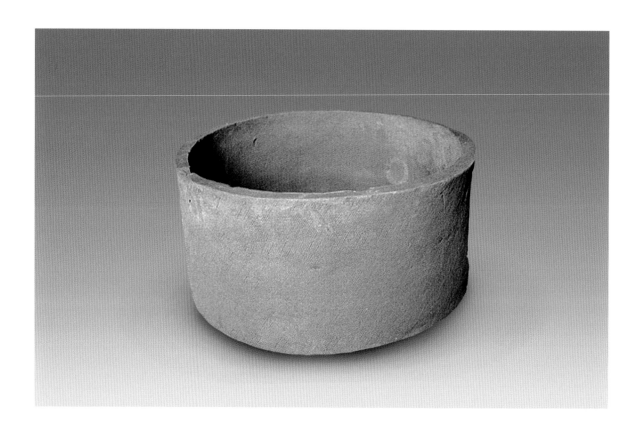

窨井圈

秦

陶质

直径 69 厘米，高 33.5 厘米

Walling of Cellar Well

Qin Dynasty

Pottery

Diameter 69 cm/ Height 33.5 cm

圈于冷藏窖井壁内。陕西咸阳秦宫一号遗址
出土。

陕西医史博物馆藏

This utensil was installed on the interior wall
of the cellar well used for cold storage. It was
excavated from No.1 Site of Qin Palace in
Xianyang City, Shaanxi Province.
Preserved in Shaanxi Museum of Medical History

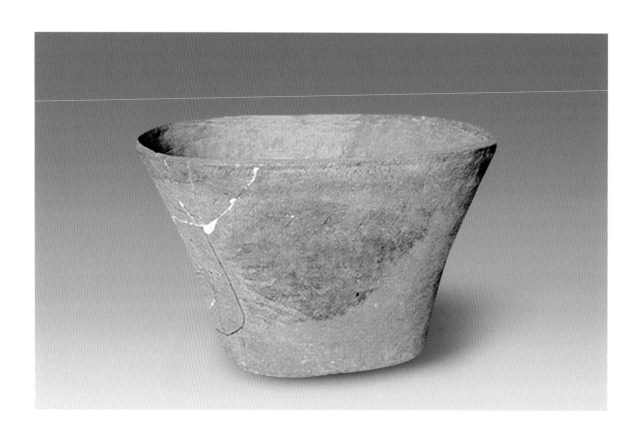

窖底盆

秦

灰陶质

上口径 100 厘米，底径 62 厘米，高 64 厘米

Cellar Basin

Qin Dynasty

Grey Pottery

Mouth Diameter 100 cm/ Bottom Diameter 62 cm/ Height 64 cm

该藏系秦咸阳宫冷藏肉类的容器，安装于 13 米深的冷藏窖井的最下面，是汉时重要的冷藏设施。

陕西医史博物馆藏

Used as a cold storage vessel for meat in Xianyang Palace of the Qin Dynasty, this utensil was installed on the bottom of the 13 meter deep cellar well. It was an important cold storage facility in the Han Dynasty.

Preserved in Shaanxi Museum of Medical History

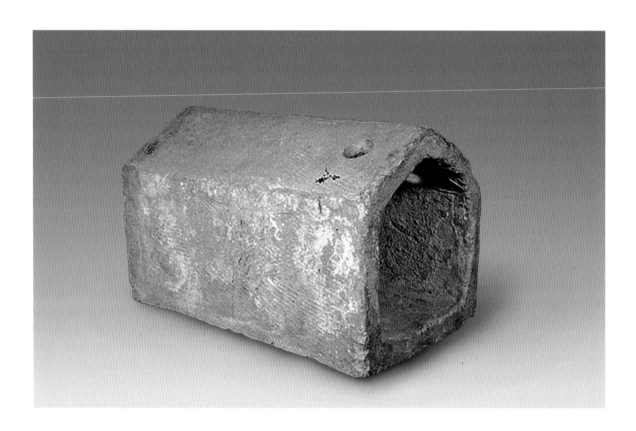

阿房宫下水道管

秦

灰陶质

长 66 厘米，高 41 厘米，壁厚 5 厘米，壁孔直径 5.9 厘米

Drainpipe of Epang Palace

Qin Dynasty

Grey Pottery

Length 66 cm/ Height 41 cm/ Wall Thickness 5 cm/ Perforation Diameter 5.9 cm

横剖面呈五角形，上部呈三角形，一侧有小圆孔。设计合理。为秦阿房宫的污水排放设施。陕西咸阳阿房宫遗址出土。

中国医史博物馆藏

With the cross section of the drainpipe in the shape of a pentagon and the top a triangle, this utensil is reasonably designed with a small round hole on one side of the top. The drainpipe, a sewage disposal facility in Qin Epang Palace, was excavated from the ruins of Epang Palace of Xianyang City, Shaanxi Province.

Preserved in Chinese Medical History Museum

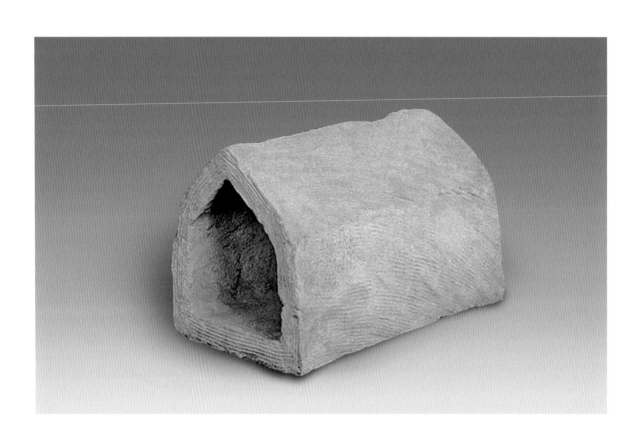

五角水道

秦

灰陶质

长 65.5 厘米，宽 42 厘米，高 46 厘米

形制同阿房宫下水管道，系秦咸阳宫中多种地下排水管道中最多的一种。

陕西医史博物馆藏

Pentagonal Water Conduit

Qin Dynasty

Grey Pottery

Length 65.5 cm/ Width 42 cm/ Height 46 cm

With the same shape and structure as the sewage pipe of Epang Palace, this kind of water pipe is most commonly used among various underdrainage pipes of Qin Xianyang Palace.

Preserved in Shaanxi Museum of Medical History

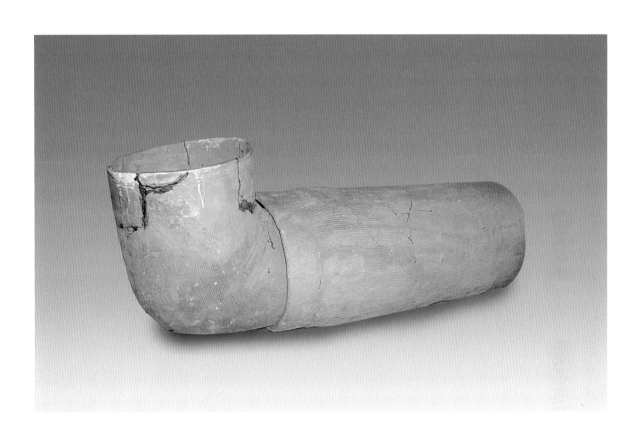

圆形陶水道

秦

灰陶质

全长37.8厘米，口沿内径17厘米，外径22厘米，
重1250克

子母口，一头口沿略大于另一端口沿，周身饰以
长条纹。完整无损。通、排水管道。陕西省咸阳
市征集。

陕西医史博物馆藏

Circular Water Conduit

Qin Dynasty

Grey Pottery

Length 37.8 cm/ Inner Mouth Diameter 17 cm/
Outer Diameter 22 cm/ Weight 1,250 g

With a snap lid and long stripe patterns all over the
body, this water pipe has one mouth rim slightly
larger than the other. The pipe was used as drain
line, and remains intact. It was collected from
Xianyang City, Shaanxi Province.

Preserved in Shaanxi Museum of Medical History

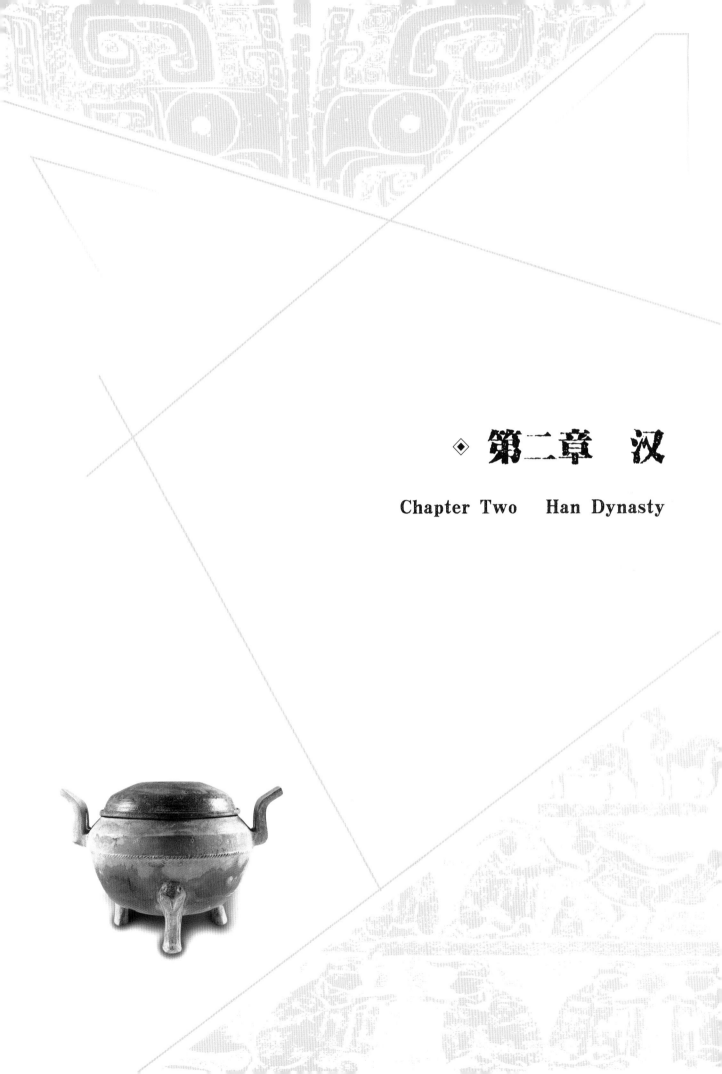

◆ 第二章　汉

Chapter Two　Han Dynasty

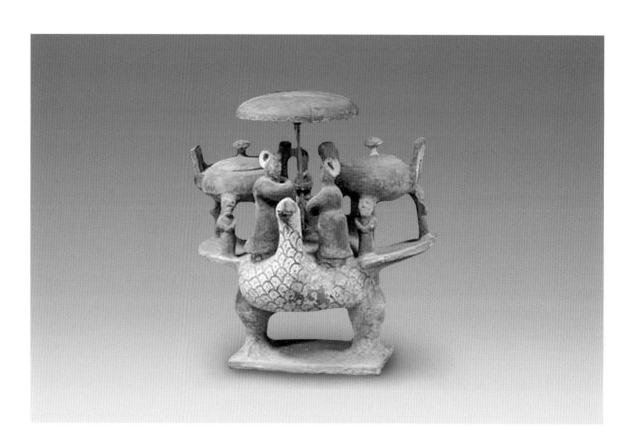

彩绘陶负鼎鸠

西汉

灰陶质

通高 53.5 厘米

Colored Pottery Turtledove Carrying Tripods

Western Han Dynasty

Grey Pottery

Height 53.5 cm

泥质灰陶。鸠鸟昂首站立，体态肥硕，双翼伸展，各负一朱绘陶鼎，背部立有三人，二人身着红袍，拱手对立，后一人身着赭色袍，双手撑伞。鸠鸟作欲飞状。鸠为吉祥之鸟，满鼎美食，供人食用，可以长生不老。彩绘陶负鼎鸠、负壶鸠、乐绣杂俑及车马俑等同时出土，造型新颖，重点突出，气势雄威，为我国汉代陶塑艺术珍品。1969 年济南市无影山出土。

济南市博物馆藏

The turtledove, an auspicious bird, stands erect and proud. It is stout and its two wings are stretching out, which carry respectively a painted tripod full of delicious food by legend that could make people immortal. There are also three people standing on the back of the turtledove. Two people in red robes standing face to face are bowing to each, while the third one in ochre robe is standing at the back with his hand holding an umbrella. At the same time, some other painted potteries were unearthed at Wuying Mountain in Jinan in 1969, all of which were novel in model and were made with the focal points standing out. They were all the precious handcrafts of pottery art in Han Dynasty.

Preserved in Jinan City Museum

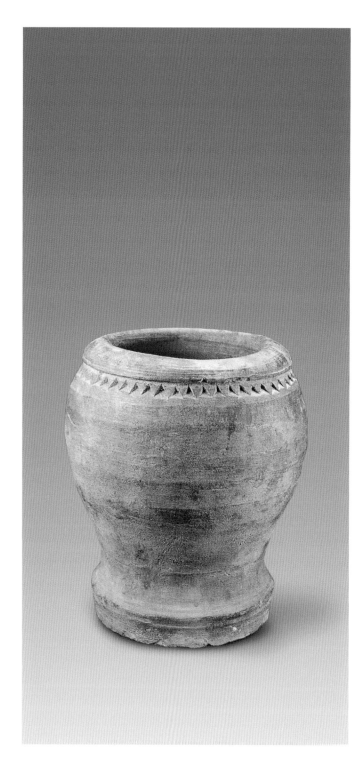

陶臼

西汉

陶质

口径 7.3 厘米，底径 8.7 厘米，腹围 36.5 厘米，高 13.4 厘米

Pottery Mortar

Western Han Dynasty

Pottery

Mouth Diameter 7.3 cm/ Bottom Diameter 8.7 cm/ Belly Perimeter 36.5 cm/ Height 13.4 cm

壁、底厚，口沿有牙状纹饰。1992 年于陕西
咸阳采集。

陕西医史博物馆藏

With a thick wall and bottom, the mortar is
decorated with tooth-shaped patterns along
the rim. It was collected from Xianyang City,
Shaanxi Province, in the year 1992.

Preserved in Shaanxi Museum of Medical History

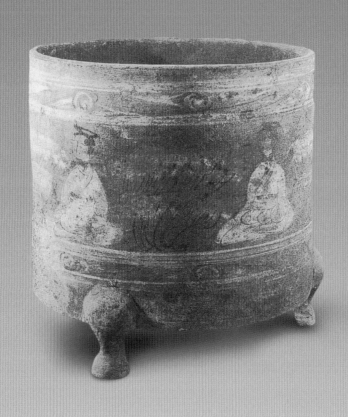

彩绘行气入静图陶奁

西汉

泥质灰陶

口径 20.2 厘米，高 19.5 厘米

彩绘行气入静图见于陶奁的腹部，用黑、红、白颜色绘成。图中五个女子席地而坐，其中一位伸长双臂，做行气之状。由其姿势和神情看，反映的正是行气入静的情景。1963 年河南洛阳出土。

洛阳博物馆藏

Painted Pottery Case with Meditating Design

Western Han Dynasty

Grey Clay Pottery

Mouth Diameter 20.2 cm/ Height 19.5 cm

The depiction of promoting the circulation of Qi and reaching the state of meditation can be found around the abdomen of the pottery case in black, red and white colours. There are five ladies sitting on the ground, one of whom stretching the arms in front of her body to gently promote the circulation of Qi. Her posture and facial expression are clear reflections of the soothing state of meditation. It was excavated from Luoyang City, Henan Province, in the year 1963.

Preserved in Luoyang Museum

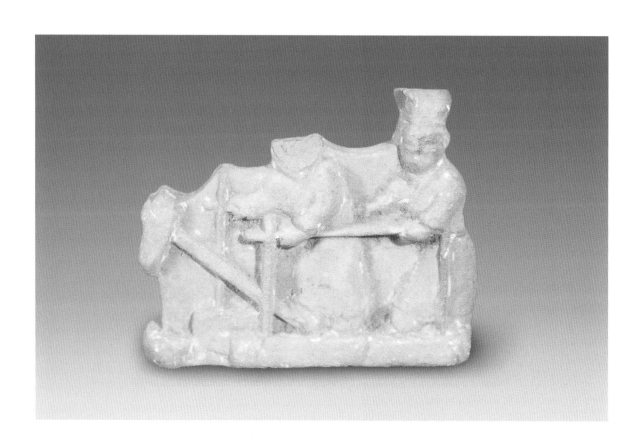

碓粮陶塑（明器）

西汉

陶质

长 15 厘米，高 15 厘米

碓亦可用于加工药物。

中国医史博物馆藏

Pottery Sculpture of Hulling Rice with Tilt Hammer (Burial Object)

Western Han Dynasty

Pottery

Length 15 cm/ Height 15 cm

The treadle-operated tilt hammer can also be used in producing medicine.

Preserved in the Chinese Medical Museum

黄釉陶仓（明器）

西汉

釉陶质

口径 5.5 厘米，底径 23 厘米，高 24 厘米

陶仓有三足，有瓦面形仓顶。于陕西咸

阳窑店采集。

陕西医史博物馆藏

Yellow-glazed Pottery Granary (Burial Object)

Western Han Dynasty

Glazed Pottery

Mouth Diameter 5.5 cm/ Bottom Diameter

23 cm/ Height 24 cm

This granary has three feet and a tile-

covered roof. It was collected from Yaodian

of Xianyang City, Shaanxi Province.

Preserved in Shaanxi Museum of Medical

History

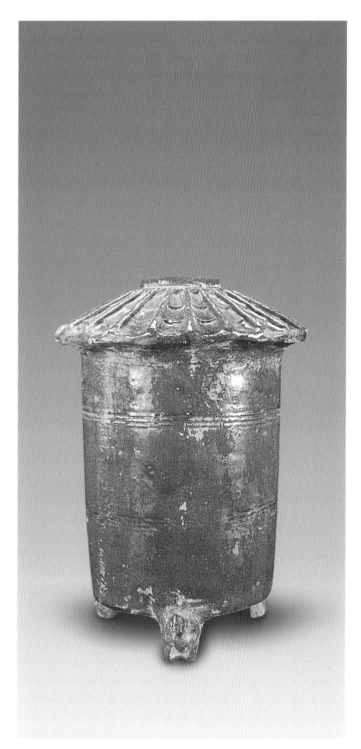

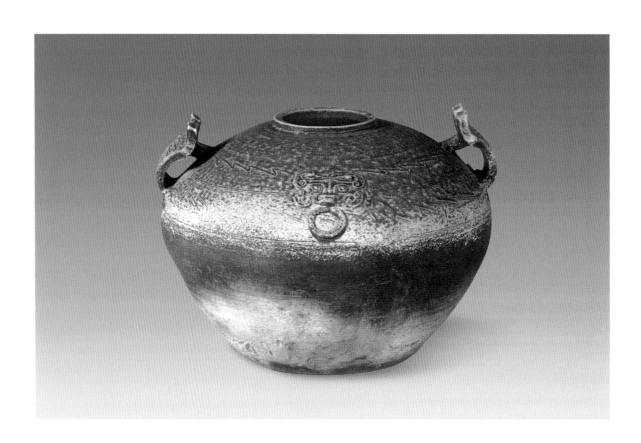

青釉陶瓿

西汉

陶质

口径 10 厘米，底径 17.3 厘米，高 23 厘米

Celadon Pottery Vessel in the Shape of Bowl

Western Han Dynasty

Pottery

Mouth Diameter 10 cm/ Bottom Diameter 17.3 cm/ Height 23 cm

瓿方唇敛口，弧肩，扁球腹，微显折腰，平底内凹。肩部置对称方耳。耳面模印兽面纹，两耳之间对称贴饰模印的兽面衔环。肩划 3 组弦纹间两道水波纹。灰褐色胎，施半截青绿色釉。该瓿的铺首衔环贴于两耳之间，有别于一般的汉代陶瓿贴饰于双耳之下，较为少见。1981 年扬州市农业科学研究所出土。

扬州博物馆藏

This vessel has a contracted mouth with a square rim, an arc-shaped shoulder, an oblate spheroid abdomen, a slightly angular waist and a flat but inwards-concave bottom. Two square ears are disposed symmetrically on the shoulder. The surface of the ear is mould-impressed with an animal mask. Between the ears are two rings suspended from an animal mask and pasted symmetrically on the sides of the vessel. Double waviness ripple patterns are carved among three sets of raised horizontal lines on the shoulder. The vase has a greyish-brown body and is half celadon-glazed. The animal mask appliqués of this vase are pasted between the two ears, which is rare and different from other pottery vessels of Han Dynasty which usually have the appliqué placed under the two ears. The object was unearthed by Yangzhou Municipal Academy of Agricultural Sciences in the year 1981.
Preserved in Yangzhou Museum

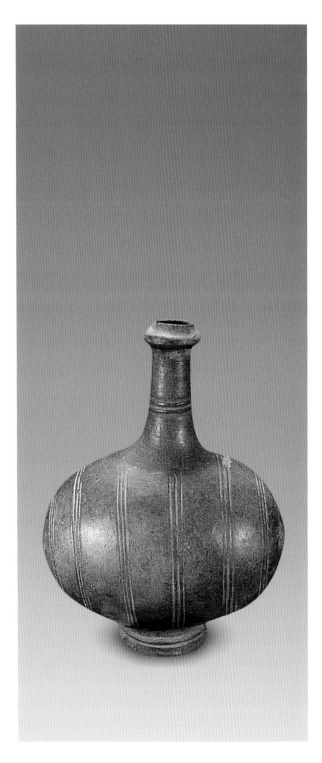

长颈鸭蛋壶

西汉

灰白陶质

口径 2.2 厘米，足径 6 厘米，颈长 7 厘米，足
高 1.5 厘米，通高 20 厘米

Oval-shaped Pot with Long Neck

Western Han Dynasty

Greyish-white Pottery

Mouth Diameter 2.2 cm/ Foot Diameter 6 cm/
Length of the Neck 7 cm/ Height of the Foot
1.5 cm/ Height 20 cm

腹呈鸭蛋形，整体表面光洁，是一件造型罕见的盛酒器。1992 年于陕西白水史官乡采集。

陕西医史博物馆藏

This pot is a wine container with an oval-shaped belly and smooth and bright surface. Such a well-designed wine container is very rare. It was collected from Shiguan Town in Baishui County, Shaanxi Province, in the year 1992.

Preserved in Shaanxi Museum of Medical History

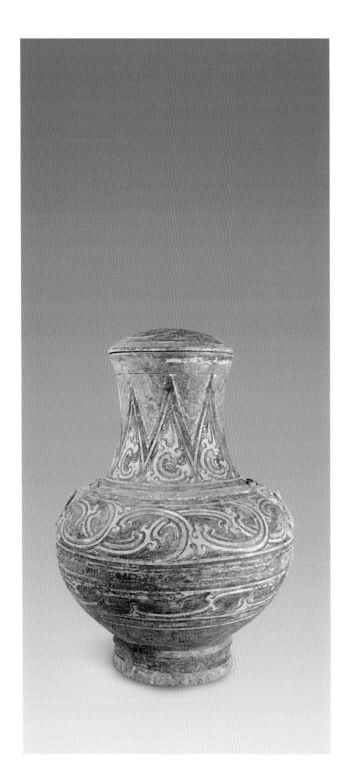

彩绘陶壶

西汉中期

灰陶质

口径 18.5 厘米，底径 19.2 厘米，通高 49.4 厘米

Painted Pottery Pot

Mid Western Han Dynasty

Grey Pottery

Mouth Diameter 18.5 cm/ Bottom Diameter

19.2 cm/ Height 49.4 cm

陶壶用泥质灰陶轮制而成，并模制出一对兽头衔环对称贴塑于壶腹两侧。口部微外敞，颈部粗壮而挺拔，腹线圆鼓，腹下是外撇的圈足，圈足表面装饰有一周凸棱。壶口上有浅钵式盒相扣。河南省济源市轵国故城桐花沟墓地出土。

河南省文物考古研究院藏

The grey pottery pot is made on a rotating wheel. Two animal heads, with rings in their mouths, are moulded symmetrically on the flanks of its belly. It has a slightly flared mouth, a thick and straight neck, a globular body and a splayed ring foot, on which is embellished a circle of raised ridge line. Its mouth is covered with a lid in the shape of a shallow "Bo" (bowl). It was unearthed from the Tonghuagou tomb in the ancient city of Zhi State, Jiyuan City, Henan Province.

Preserved in Henan Provincial Institute of Cultural Heritage and Archaeology

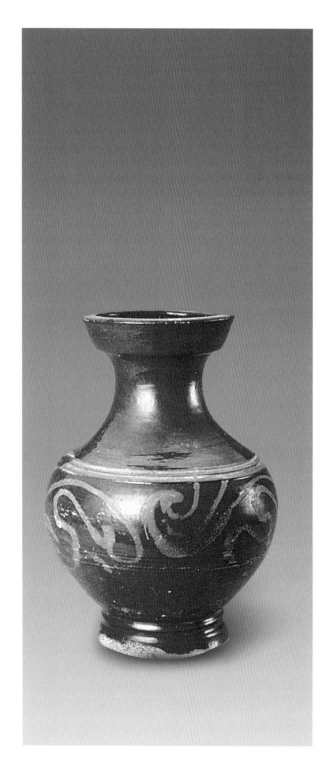

褐红釉加彩壶

西汉晚期

釉陶质

口径 15.2 厘米，底径 13.6 厘米，高 32 厘米

Painted Pot with Brownish-red Glaze

Late Western Han Dynasty

Glazed Pottery

Mouth Diameter 15.2 cm/ Bottom Diameter 13.6 cm/

Height 32 cm

壶方唇盘口，浑圆的腹部下接外撇的圈足，线条饱满圆润。器表满布深红色釉，釉面匀称光洁，明亮如新。肩部和下腹部各饰有两周凹弦纹，且上组凹弦纹内另加绿釉填充，两组弦纹之间为几组绿釉勾连状卷云纹。陕西省宝鸡市谭家村四号墓出土。

北京大学赛克勒考古与艺术博物馆藏

This finely painted pot has a dish-shaped mouth with a thick lip, a globular body and a spreading ring foot. It is fully and evenly covered with crimson glaze, which looks bright and clean. Its shoulder and the lower part of its belly are decorated with two circles of concave bow string patterns respectively, in between which are several green-glazed interlocking designs in the shape of rolling clouds. The inside of the concave bowstring patterns on the shoulder is also filled with green glaze. The pot was unearthed from No.4 Tomb in Tanjia Village of Baoji City, Shaanxi Province.

Preserved in Arthur M. Sackler Museum of Art and Archeology at Peking University

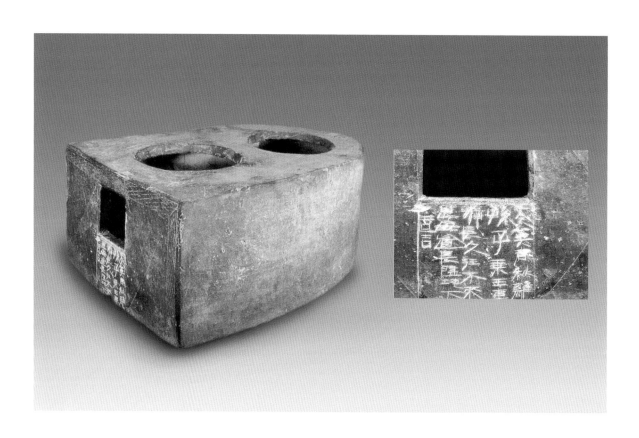

陶灶（明器）

西汉

陶质

长 26 厘米，高 11.5 厘米

灶口：高 4.2 厘米，宽 4.6 厘米

Pottery Stove (Burial Object)

Western Han Dynasty

Pottery

Length 26 cm/ Height 11.5 cm

The Stove Opening: Height 4.2 cm/ Width 4.6 cm

灶口下有 5 行 27 字铭文："大人弃春秋，离子孙，乘王车游，长久往不来，甚（慎）毋置，长随地下，□造，吉。"藏品为明器，1978 年于陕西眉县采集。

陕西医史博物馆藏

An inscriptions of twenty-seven characters in five lines are carved under the stove opening. It served as a burial object, and was collected in Meixian County, Shaanxi Province, in the year 1978.

Preserved in Shaanxi Museum of Medical History

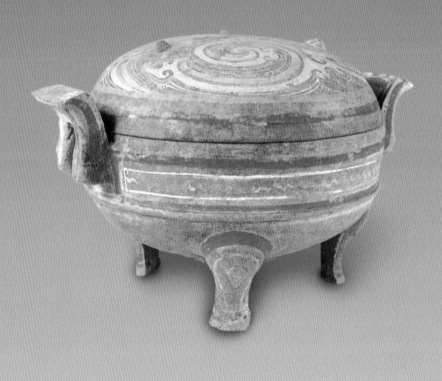

彩绘陶鼎

西汉中期

陶质

通宽 22 厘米，通高 15.8 厘米

鼎为深色细腻之泥质灰陶质。整体造型矮胖浑圆，彩绘装饰繁简有致，布局得当。如此具有高度艺术水平的彩绘且保留完好如新的陶器，在已发掘的汉代文物中尚属罕见，诚为不可多得的艺术珍品。河南省济源市轵国故城桐花沟墓地出土。

河南省文物考古研究院藏

Painted Pottery "Ding" (Tripod)

Mid Western Han Dynasty

Pottery

Width 22 cm/ Height 15.8 cm

This "Ding", with a compressed globular body, is of dark grey clay pottery with fine texture. The painted decorations on the "Ding" are well balanced. It is very rare and of high value in the unearthed cultural relics of the Han Dynasty for its high artistic level of coloured drawings and its excellent state of preservation which makes its appearance new. The object was unearthed from a tomb at Tonghuagou in the ancient city of Zhi State in Jiyuan City, Henan Province.

Preserved in Henan Provincial Institute of Cultural Heritage and Archaeology

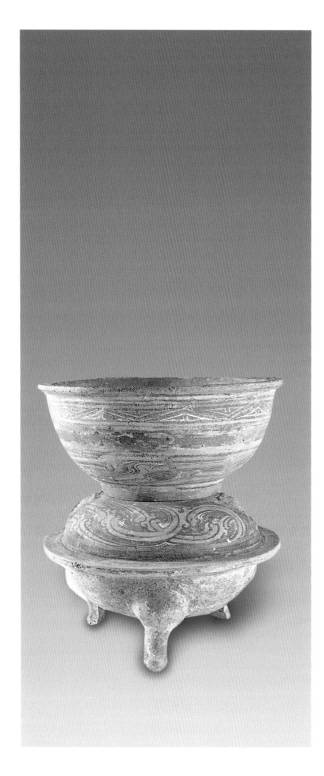

彩绘陶甗

西汉中期

陶质

甗口径 21 厘米，高 9.5 厘米；鼎腹径 18 厘米，

通高 22.6 厘米

Painted Pottery "Yan" (Steamer)

Mid Western Han Dynasty

Pottery

Mouth Diameter 21 cm/ Height of Upper Part 9.5 cm/

Belly Diameter of the Tripod 18 cm/ Height 22.6 cm

上部是方唇敞口的甑，底面有几个长条形镂孔而形成箅子，其下是较矮的圈足；下部是敛口鼓腹的鼎，鼎口稍小并直立，因而能套入甑的圈足内，使来自鼎内的蒸汽顺畅涌入甑而不致过多地外泄。鼎腹有一周宽平沿，腹下 3 条蹄足。造型与用色均甚为和谐。复合炊具。河南省济源市轵国故城桐花沟墓地出土。

河南省文物考古研究院藏

The upper part of the vessel is a "Zeng" (steamer) with a trumpet mouth and a galleried mouth rim. On the bottom of the "Zeng" are several long and narrow holes which form a grate. The "Zeng" has a relatively short ring foot, which stands on the lower part, "Ding" (tripod). This "Ding" has a rounded belly and an upright inverted rim, which can be nested into the Zeng's ring foot, for it is a little smaller than the ring foot. This structure allows steam to go smoothly from the "Ding" to the "Zeng" without leaking. On the belly of the "Ding" is a circle of wide and flat flange, and under its belly are three horseshoe-shaped feet. It is a compound cooker harmoniously shaped and was coloured and unearthed from a tomb at Tonghuagou in an ancient city of the Zhi State, Jiyuan City, Henan Province.

Preserved in Henan Provincial Institute of Cultural Heritage and Archaeology

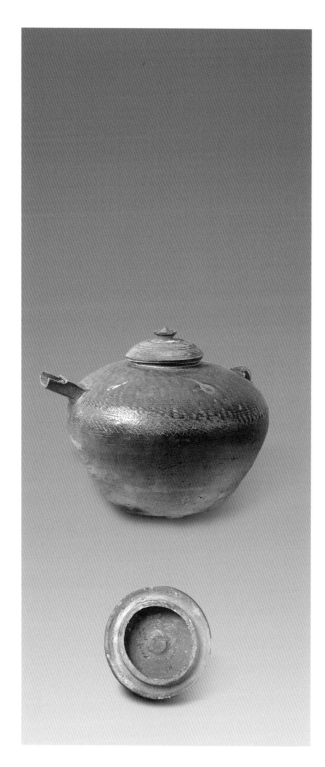

青釉陶钟

西汉

釉陶质

口径 13.8 厘米，腹径 41.4 厘米，底径 22 厘米，

高 33.4 厘米

Celadon-glazed Pottery Pot

Western Han Dynasty

Glazed Pottery

Mouth Diameter 13.8 cm/ Belly Diameter 41.4 cm/

Bottom Diameter 22 cm/ Height 33.4 cm

陶钟带盖、盖上为蘑菇状纽，盖缘内侧有一周凹槽，合于口之上，盖面刻有弦纹，盖内墨书"锺盖"两字。器身方唇，束颈，圆肩，鼓腹，平底。下有三扁矮足。肩一侧为一蕉叶纹半环耳，耳两侧各有两个弦纹贴饰，肩的另一侧为铲形流，上刻有斜格纹，腹中部有网纹一周，肩及上腹部有三周水波纹，间以弦纹，胎色灰白，通体施青褐色釉。此锺造型独特，硕大浑厚，殊为少见。1989年江苏省仪征市新集镇团山出土。

仪征博物馆藏

This pot has a lid with a mushroom-shaped knob. Along the inner edge of the lid is a ring of concave groove, making the lid and the mouth fit well. The lid surface is incised with bowstring patterns. On the interior of the lid are written two Chinese characters "Zhong Gai" (the lid of the pot) with ink. The pot has a galleried mouth, a short waisted neck, a rounded shoulder, a globular body, a flat bottom, and three flat and short feet. On one side of the shoulder is a half ring-like ear with a banana leaf pattern, and the sides of the ear are decorated with two bowstring patterns respectively. On the other side of the shoulder is a spade-shaped spout with skew lattice patterns on. The middle part of the belly is incised with a ring of net-like patterns, while the shoulder and the upper part of the belly are decorated with three rings of ripple patterns, which alternate with bowstring patterns. The greyish-white body is covered with bluish-brown glaze. The uniquely-designed pot with such a huge size is rarely seen. This collection was unearthed from the Xinji Town, Tuan mountain in Yizheng city, Jiangsu Province, in the year 1989. Preserved in Yizheng Museum

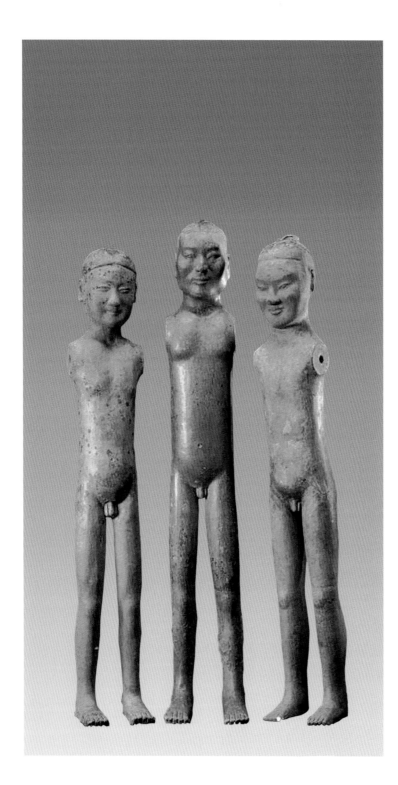

彩绘着衣式木臂男俑

西汉

陶质

高 58~62 厘米

Painted Male Figures in Dress

Western Han Dynasty

Pottery

Height 58~ 62 cm

俑为裸体。通体施有橙红色彩绘，头发、须眉、瞳仁、鼻孔、耳、肚脐、生殖器官等人体九窍无一不备。陶俑原本安装有木质的手臂，身穿丝质或麻质的战袍，外穿皮质的铠甲，因长期埋于地下，导致衣物腐朽、木臂成灰，发掘时以裸体缺臂的状态面世。

汉阳陵博物馆藏

The figurines are naked and entirely painted in reddish-orange. They are modelled with all nine orifices, including hairs, beard, eyebrows, pupils, nostrils, ears, navels and reproductive organs.The pottery figurines had been fitted wooden arms and dressed in silken or linen war robes under the leather armors. They have been buried underground over such a long period that the clothing has rotted away and the arms have turned into ash. The figurines were excavated naked and armless.

Preserved in Hanyangling Museum

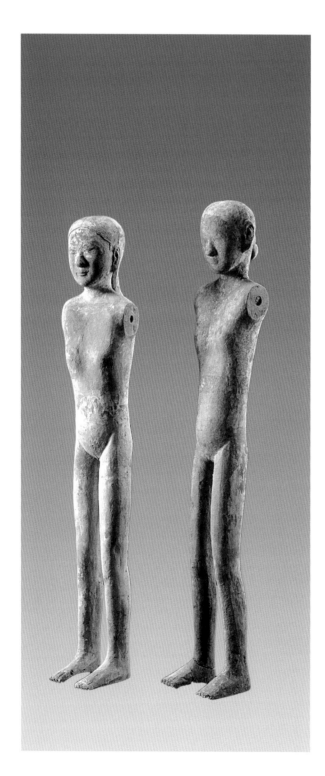

彩绘着衣式木臂女俑

西汉

陶质

左高 52.5 厘米，右高 55 厘米

Painted Female Figures in Dress

West Han Dynasty

Pottery

Left: Height 52.5 cm; Right: Height 55 cm

俑为裸体。通体彩绘，头发、鼻孔、耳、生
殖器官等人体九窍刻画细腻。因长埋于地下，
导致所着衣物腐朽、木臂成灰，发掘时以裸
体缺臂的状态面世。

咸阳市文物保护中心藏

The figurines are naked and entirely painted.
Their nine orifices are delicately modelled, such
as hairs, nostrils, ears, reproductive organs and
the like. They have been buried underground
over such a long period that the clothing has
rotted away and the arms have turned into
ash. The figurines were excavated naked and
armless.

Preserved in Xianyang Cultural Relics Conservation
Centre

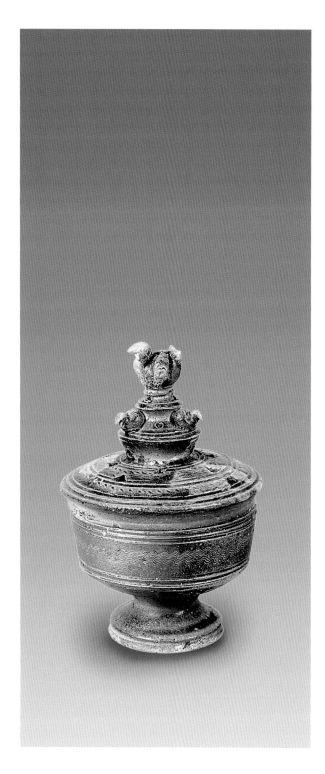

青釉陶薰

西汉

釉陶质

口径 9.6 厘米，腹径 12.4 厘米，底径 7.5 厘米，
高 19.1 厘米

Greenish-brown-glazed Censer

Western Han Dynasty

Glazed Pottery

Mouth Diameter 9.6 cm/ Belly Diameter 12.4 cm/

Bottom Diameter 7.5 cm/ Height 19.1 cm

盖顶中部凸起一棱柱，顶端上立一鸟，鸟身中部有一透孔，鸟作振翅欲飞状。棱柱外缘立三小鸟，柱身有 9 个透孔。盖面上有 8 个三角形镂孔，上刻人字篦点纹 5 道，弦纹 2 道。器身作子母口，深腹，下腹斜折，倒置豆形足，腹外壁饰一周水波汶，材质坚致，通体施青褐色釉，釉面光滑。1994 年江苏省仪征市刘集镇联营村赵庄出土。

仪征博物馆藏

On the centre of the lid stands a prism with a rousant bird on its top and a hole in the middle of the bird's body. Around the rim of the prism stand three birds. On the prism nine holes can be found. On the surface of the lid are eight triangle holes incised with five comb patterns in the shape of a Chinese-character " 人 " (Ren) and two rips of string patterns. The body is designed to be a snap lid. The censer has a deep belly, the lower belly tapering to an upturned bean-shaped foot. The exterior wall of the belly is decorated with a tier of ripple patterns. The hard body of the censer is covered with bright and smooth greenish-brown glaze. The collection was unearthed at Zhaozhuang, Lianying Village, Liuji Town, Yizheng City, Jiangsu Province, in the year 1994. Preserved in Yizheng Museum

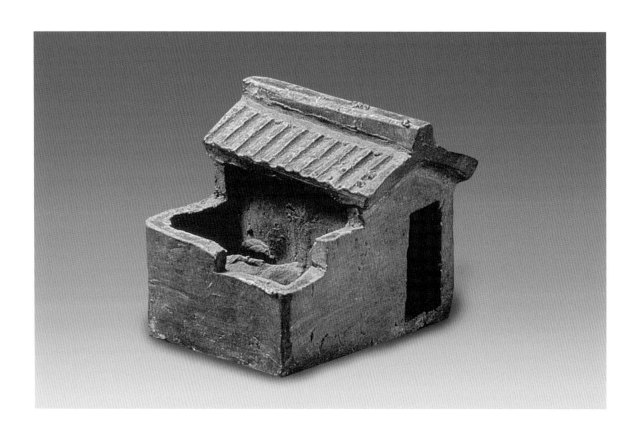

釉陶连猪圈式厕所

西汉

釉陶质

面宽 7 厘米，进深 5.5 厘米，高 9 厘米

Glazed Pottery Toilet with Pigsty Latrine

Western Han Dynasty

Glazed Pottery

Width 7 cm/ Depth 5.5 cm/ Height 9 cm

此器由厕所和猪圈两部分组成。厕所为硬山式房屋，屋顶出檐，刻有瓦珑。在一侧山墙单开门，厕所内有蹲坑，蹲坑旁的墙脚处开有粪便的出洞。在另侧山墙及后檐的上部均有三个出气孔。猪圈依厕所墙而建，另三面围有矮墙，猪圈内有一陶猪，依猪食槽而立。猪圈和厕所连在一起表示当时已注意积肥用于农业生产。南京市溧水区渔歌乡仓口村富家山西汉墓出土。

南京市溧水区博物馆藏

This object is composed of the toilet and the pigsty. The toilet with the Chinese flush-gabled roof has the eaves decorated with sea clam pattern. On one side of the gable wall of the toilet is a single-leaf door. In the toilet is a squatting pot by the side of a hole for feces in the corner. On the other side of the gable wall and the upper part of the back eaves are three vent holes respectively. The pigsty is surrounded by parapets on three sides and the toilet on the other, with a pottery pig standing by the trough in it. The structure of the pigsty next to the latrine shows that people at that time were aware of collecting manure for the agricultural use. This collection was excavated from the tomb of the Western Han Dynasty in Fujia Mountain of Cangkou Village in Yuge Township of Lishui District, in Nanjing City.

Preserved in Lishui County Museum, Nanjing City

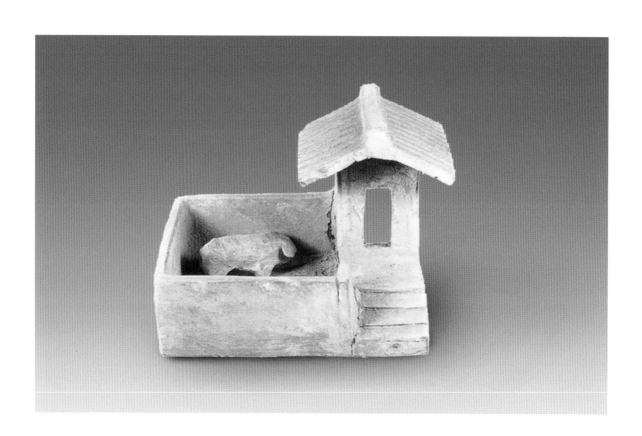

陶猪圈

西汉

陶质

边长 18 厘米，高 17 厘米

Pottery Pigsty

Western Han Dynasty

Pottery

Length 18 cm/ Height 17 cm

猪圈方形，与厕所相连，圈内有陶猪一只。
明器。河南郑州郊区出土。

上海中医药博物馆藏

With a pottery pig in it, the square pigsty is next
to a toilet. It served as a burial object, and was
unearthed from the suburbs of Zhengzhou City,
Henan Province.
Preserved in Shanghai Museum of Traditional
Chinese Medicine

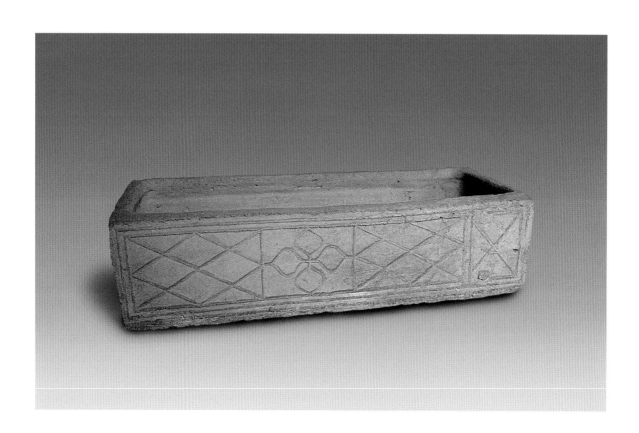

陶棺

西汉

陶质

长 79 厘米，宽 29.5 厘米，高 20 厘米

Pottery Coffin

Western Han Dynasty

Pottery

Length 79 cm/ Width 29.5 cm/ Height 20 cm

陶棺两侧有相同纹饰。该藏为用于小孩的葬具。

陕西咸阳北原出土。

陕西医史博物馆藏

On both sides of the coffin are carved the same patterns. It served as a burial object for kid, and was excavated from Beiyuan of Xianyang City, Shaanxi Province.

Preserved in Shaanxi Museum of Medical History

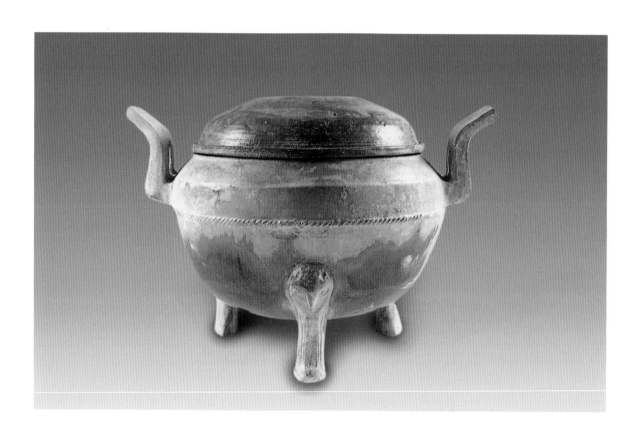

釉陶鼎

西汉晚期

釉陶质

口径 12.1 厘米，通高 18 厘米

Glazed Pottery "Ding" (Tripod)

Late Western Han Dynasty

Glazed Pottery

Mouth Diameter 12.1 cm/ Height 18 cm

此鼎口扣合一个平底盘式盖，从而与鼎身形成浑圆的球形曲线，饱满而圆润。由于胎质细密且釉层均匀，釉面光洁如镜，加之釉面上细微的开片纹犹如冰乍玉裂，造就了一种既明亮又朦胧的意境。而釉层的严重返铅，使光照下的釉面既有丝丝银毫，又富层层光晕，流光溢彩。河南省济源市轵国故城泗涧沟墓地出土。

河南省文物考古研究院藏

This "Ding", covered with a lid in the shape of a flat-bottomed dish, looks plump and mellow, for the unique shape of the lid forms a round spherical curve together with the body of the "Ding". With fine body texture and even enamel layer, the "Ding" is shining like a mirror. The glaze with small crackles resembles cracked ice or jade, looking bright and hazy. The reemergence of lead in the glaze makes the enamel layer shining and lustrous with silvery hair and layers of haloes. The collection was unearthed from a tomb at Sijiangou in the ancient city of Zhi State, Jiyuan City, Henan Province.

Preserved in Henan Provincial Institute of Cultural Heritage and Archaeology

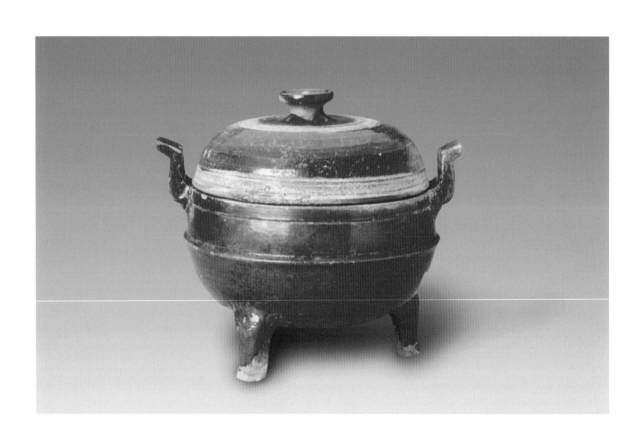

褐红釉加彩陶鼎

西汉晚期

釉陶质

口径 19.1 厘米，高 21 厘米

Pottery "Ding" (Tripod) with Brownish-red Glaze

Late Western Han Dynasty

Glazed Pottery

Mouth Diameter 19.1 cm/ Height 21 cm

此鼎把手周围及鼎盖口部各有一周绿彩装饰带，绿彩之下，有模印的菱形格纹若隐若现。整个器物满施褐红色釉。这种复合彩釉的装饰技法，代表了两汉时期釉陶装饰工艺的最高水平。陕西省宝鸡市谭家村四号墓出土。

北京大学赛克勒考古与艺术博物馆藏

Around the handles and the lid rim is a ornamental band of green painting, under which stamped rhombus designs can be gleamingly seen. This "Ding" is fully coated with brownish-red glaze. The approach of decoration with multiple coloured glazes represents the top level of the craftsmanship of glazed pottery decoration in the Han Dynasty. The collection was unearthed from No.4 Tomb in Tanjia Village, Baoji City, Shaanxi Province.

Preserved in Arthur M. Sackler Museum of Art and Archeology of Peking University

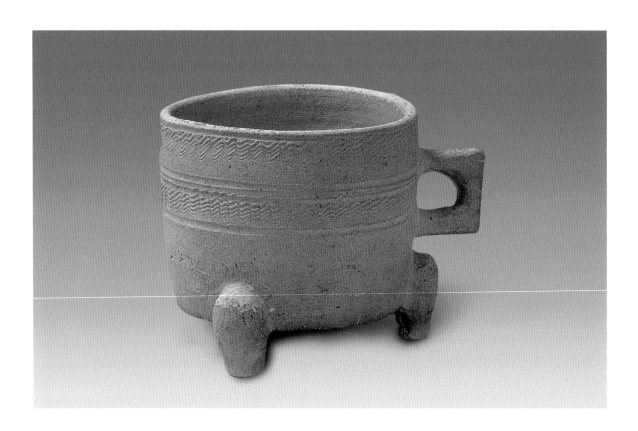

三足硬陶把杯

西汉

陶质

口径 11.2 厘米，底径 10 厘米，通高 9.8 厘米

Tripod Hard Pottery Cup with Handle

Western Han Dynasty

Pottery

Mouth Diameter 11.2 cm/ Bottom Diameter 10 cm/ Height 9.8 cm

三兽足，素面。杯身直筒形，侧壁装一外方内圆手柄。胎质坚硬，叩之有声。外壁罩青釉，大部剥落。口沿饰水波一道，中部饰弦纹两道及水波纹一道。把杯的整体造型粗壮有力，但加上悬空的器足和寥寥的水波纹及镂空把手，使全器显得轻巧美观。由此体现了汉代先民简约的审美情趣。

南京市博物馆藏

The unglazed cup has a straight tubular body with three beast feet. To one side of the cup is attached a handle with a square outer frame and a circular inner frame. The body is so hard that it produces a ringing sound when knocked. The exterior wall is coated with green glaze, most of which has peeled off. The mouth rim is decorated with a ring of ripple pattern, while around the stomach are two rings of string patterns and a ring of ripple pattern. The overall design of the cup is sturdy and robust, but the pendent legs, a few ripple patterns and the hollow-out handle make it lightweight and pleasing to the eye, which reflects the simple aesthetic taste of the people in the Han Dynasty. Preserved in Nanjing Museum

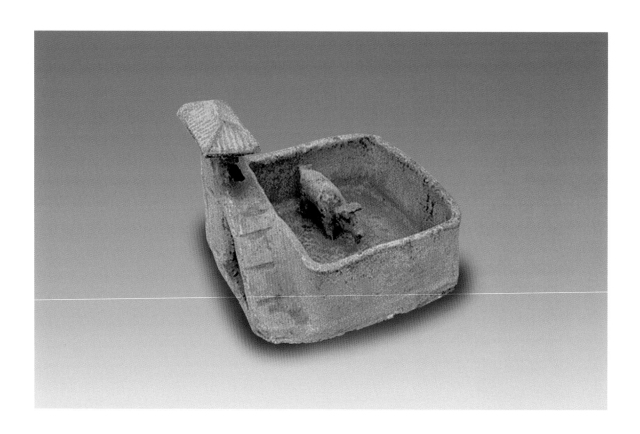

绿釉陶猪圈

西汉

陶质

底宽 24 厘米，宽 24 厘米，高 16 厘米

Green-glazed Pottery Pigsty

Western Han Dynasty

Pottery

Bottom Width 24 cm/ Width 24 cm/ Height 16 cm

猪圈方形,厕所建于猪圈上方并与猪圈相连,圈内有陶猪一只,人畜分开反映古人已经十分注意环境卫生。

北京御生堂中医药博物馆藏

The square pigsty has a pottery pig and the toilet on the top of it serves to connect with the pigsty. The separation of people and animal shows the people in Han Dynasty cared about sanitation.

Preserved in Chinese Medicine Museum of Beijing Yu Sheng Tang Drugstore

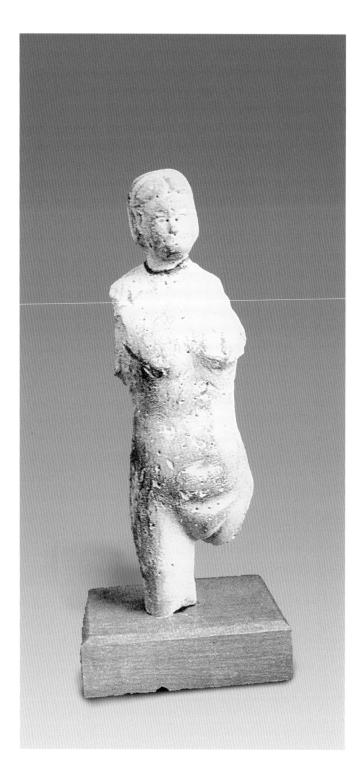

针灸陶人

东汉

陶质

残高 20 厘米

Pottery Figurine for Acupuncture and Moxibustion

Eastern Han Dynasty

Pottery

Remaining Height 20 cm

人像为裸体女性形象，分布有数十个细孔，似按经络穴位排列。河南南阳医圣祠出土。

河南南阳医圣祠藏

The object is in the form of a nude female figurine, on which are dozens of needling points regularly disposed with meridians and collaterals or acupuncture points of human body. It was unearthed from the Medical Sage Ancestral Temple, Nanyang City, Henan Province.

Presered in the Medical Sage Ancestral Temple, Nanyang City, Henan Province

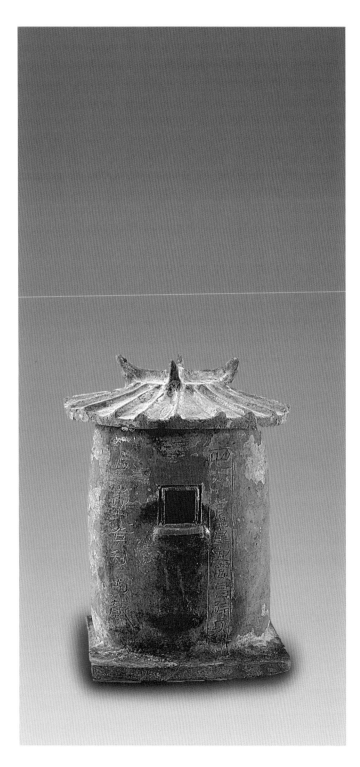

铭文绿釉陶仓

东汉

釉陶质

底长 19.8 厘米，宽 19.5 厘米，腹径
18.2 厘米，通高 29.7 厘米

Green-glazed Pottery Granary
with Inscriptions

Eastern Han Dynasty

Glazed Pottery

Bottom Length 19.8 cm/ Width 19.5 cm/

Belly Diameter 18.2 cm/ Height 29.7 cm

此器质地为红胎釉陶，分为两截，其上部为屋盖，下部为仓库。盖呈伞形状，盖屋顶为十字形屋脊，盖屋面饰有凸起的瓦垄纹。仓房呈圆筒形体，上部稍收，下部稍大，平底下置文武台座。仓房的中部安置有一窗框的单扇窗。窗的两侧各有一竖排铭文，铭文为阴文隶书，左侧铭文为："屯（囷）崇（瑞）大吉利，内（纳）谷。"右侧长方形框内铭为："屯（囷）卜鸟，名凤皇（凰），宜富昌，辟（避）央（殃）。"陶仓满施绿釉，胎釉结合不太紧密，铭文处釉较厚，釉色晶莹亮泽。1992年出土于邗江甘泉镇姚湾村顺利组。

扬州市邗江区文物管理委员会藏

This granary, consisting of a roof and a warehouse, is made of glazed pottery with red roughcast. Resembling an umbrella, the roof has a cross-shaped ridge and its surface is decorated with alternating concave and convex patterns. The cylindrical warehouse widens slightly at the bottom, and a "wen-wu" (civil and military) pedestal is located beneath its flat bottom. The middle part of the warehouse wall is decorated with a single casement window with window frames, on each side of which is an inscription written vertically, cut in intaglio. The inscription to the left reads: "Tun Rui Da Ji Li, Na Gu(Storing grains to bring good fortune and luck)". To the right is a rectangular frame with the inscription of "Tun Shang Niao, Ming Feng Huang, Yi Fu Chang, Bi Yang(Hoarding the auspicious bird phoenix to bring wealth and prosperity while avoiding misfortune)". The pottery granary is fully coated with green glaze, but the glaze and the body are not closely combined. The glaze of the inscriptions is relatively thicker and the colour transparent and glossy. The object was excavated by Shunli Team of Yaowan Village at Ganquan Town in Hanjiang City, Jiangsu Province, in the year 1992.

Preserved in the Department of Cultural Relics Conservation, Hanjiang District, Yangzhou City

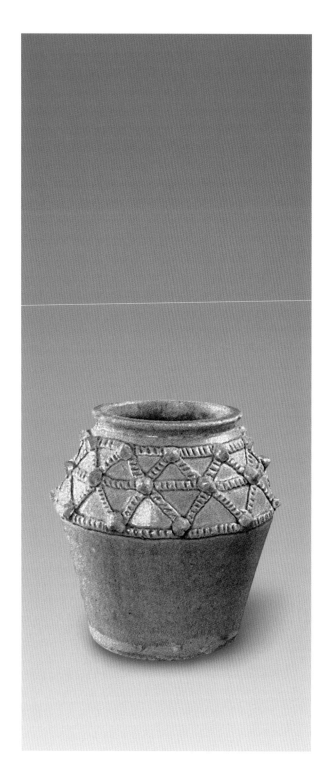

青瓷罐

东汉

瓷质

口径 11.1 厘米，高 17.6 厘米

Celadon Jar

Eastern Han Dynasty

Porcelain

Mouth Diameter 11.1 cm/ Height 17.6 cm

该罐敞口斜肩，深腹平底，胎体呈浅灰色。罐的外表满施青色釉，釉色温润亮丽，如一泓清水。肩部饰有用泥条捏塑而成的网状纹，像交叉的绳索，交叉处用尖锥状乳钉固定，形似挽扣的绳结。浙江奉化白杜东汉墓出土。

浙江省博物馆藏

The jar features a flared mouth, a sloping shoulder, a deep belly and a flat bottom. It has a light grey body coated with celadon glaze all over its exterior. The glaze is so smooth and bright that it looks like clear water. Its shoulder is decorated with netlike patterns made of clayish bars, which resemble tied cords, and the intersections are fixed by cone-shaped nails, which look like knots. The jar was unearthed from the tomb of the Eastern Han Dynasty in Baidu Town, Fenghua City, Zhejiang Province. Preserved in Zhejiang Provincial Museum

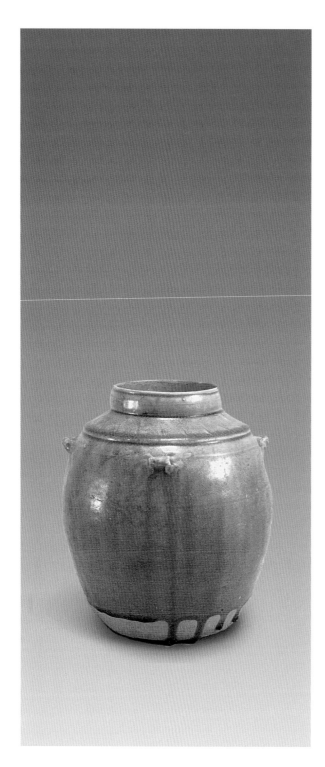

青瓷四系罐

东汉

瓷质

口径 10.8 厘米，底径 12.9 厘米，腹径 21 厘米，
通高 22.5 厘米

Green-glazed Jar with Four Rings

Eastern Han Dynasty

Porcelain

Mouth Diameter 10.8 cm/ Bottom Diameter 12.9 cm/

Belly Diameter 21 cm/ Height 22.5 cm

罐直口，圆唇内敛，短颈，弧肩微凸，鼓腹，平底内凹。肩部起一道圆脊，其下置四个对称的泥条状横系。灰白色胎上印细麻布纹，施青黄釉，底部有流釉，釉面有细开片。1980 年出土于邗江区甘泉乡香巷村东汉砖室墓中。

扬州博物馆藏

The jar has a straight mouth, a contracted mouth, a short neck, a slightly raised curving shoulder, a globular body and a concave base. On its shoulder is one round ridge, under which are placed four symmetrical horizontal rings, which resemble clayish bars. On the greyish-white body are stamped thin linen patterns. The jar is coated with bluish-yellow glaze, on whose bottom small crackles and glaze-saggings can be seen. It was unearthed from the brick-chambered tomb of the Eastern Han Dynasty in Xiangxiang Village, Ganquan Town, Hanjiang District, Jiangsu Province, in the year 1980. Preserved in Yangzhou Museum

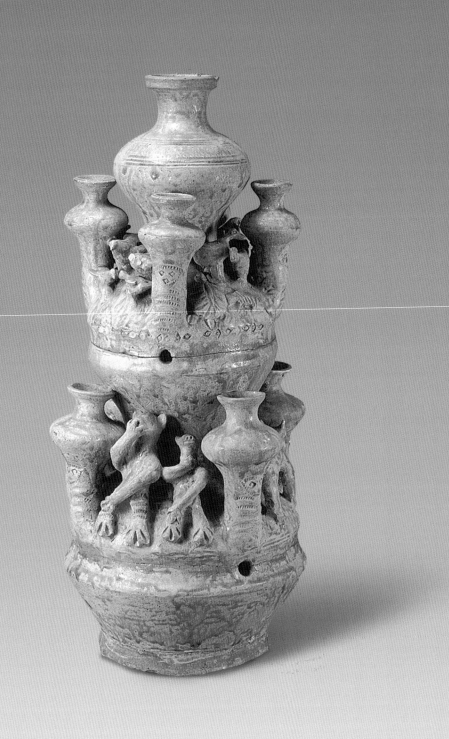

青釉堆塑九联罐

东汉

瓷质

口径 6.5 厘米，底径 16 厘米，高 50.5 厘米

胎体坚致，釉色灰青。造型为九罐相连，即由两层五联罐相接而成。顶部为一完整罐形器；上下两层均等距离围塑四个小罐，小罐下的柱面刻印怪异的人面纹，罐与罐之间堆塑鸡、鸭、猪、狗、羊、熊、鱼、鳖等各种动物。

常州博物馆藏

Celadon Jar with Nine Connecting Jars

Eastern Han Dynasty

Porcelain

Mouth Diameter 6.5 cm/ Bottom Diameter 16 cm/ Height 50.5 cm

The body of the jar is hard and compact, and is coated with celadon glaze. The jar is made up with nine connecting jars, which are arranged in two layers. Each layer has five jars connected to each other. The top of this vessel is in the shape of a single jar, below which are two layers of small jars, with four small jars on each layer equally distanced from the centre. Beneath the small jars are pillars, on which are stamped strange human-face designs. Various animal figures, such as chickens, ducks, pigs, dogs, sheep, bears, fish, and Amyda sinensis, etc. are moulded in between the small jars.

Preserved in Changzhou Museum

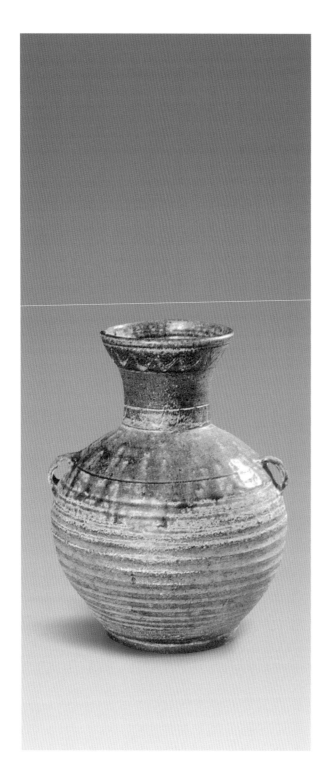

青瓷双系盘口壶

东汉

瓷质

通高 26.8 厘米

Double-handed Celadon Pot with Dish-shaped Mouth

Eastern Han Dynasty

Porcelain

Height 26.8 cm

盘口壶是指壶的颈部以上部位突起，壶口形似浅盘，是汉代尤其东汉流行的式样。此件盘口外敞，颈部粗壮，溜肩鼓腹，肩部有对称双系，腹下为假圈足式大平底。肩部以上施有青灰色釉，釉色几近黄褐色，釉层较厚。未施釉的部位胎体呈褐红色，并有平行的十周凹弦纹。口沿与肩部各饰一周水波纹，系在釉下刻画而成。山西省朔州市平朔露天煤矿出土。

山西省考古研究所藏

A pot with a dish-shaped mouth means that the part above the pot's neck expands outwards so that its mouth resembles a shallow dish. The design of the pot was popular in the Han Dynasty, especially in the Eastern Han Dynasty. This pot has a flared mouth, a thick neck, a sloping shoulder, a globular body above a bottom which seems to be a ring foot, but actually acts as a big flat bottom. There is a pair of handles on its shoulder. The part above its shoulder is coated with bluish-grey glaze which is almost tawny, with a thick enamel layer. The unglazed part of the pot exposes the pot's maroon-coloured body and is decorated with ten horizontal circles of concave bowstring patterns. Its mouth rim and shoulder are respectively embellished with a circle of ripple patterns which is carved under the glaze. The collection was unearthed from the Pingshuo open-pit coal mines in Shuozhou City, Shanxi Province.
Preserved in Shanxi Provincial Institute of Archaeology

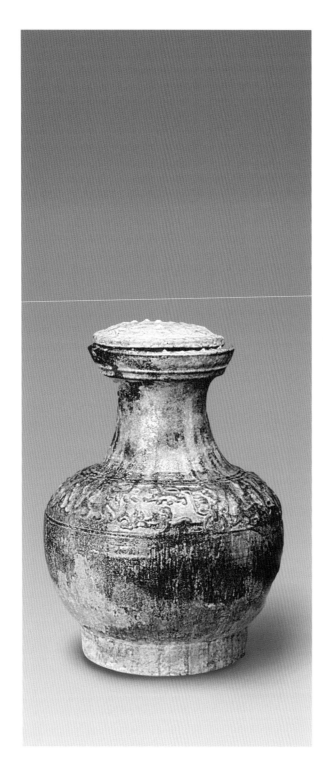

绿釉狩猎纹陶壶

东汉

釉陶质

口径 22 厘米，高 49.5 厘米

Green-glazed Pottery Pot with Hunting Scenes

Eastern Han Dynasty

Glazed Pottery

Mouth Diameter 22 cm/ Height 49.5 cm

壶为盘口，短颈，圆鼓形腹，平底，半球形盖。通体施翠绿色釉。口沿下有突起弦纹两道，肩部堆塑带状狩猎纹，两边饰铺首衔环，盖面饰卷草纹。陶壶形体硕大，制作规整，釉面光亮，表现了汉代铅釉陶器的制作水平。

山西博物院藏

The pot has a dish-shaped mouth, a short neck, a globular body, a flat bottom and a hemispheric lid. It is fully coated with emerald glaze. There are two rings of raised string patterns under its mouth rim, and on its shoulder is molded a band of hunting scenes. Animal heads with rings in their mouths are attached to the flanks of the shoulder, and rolling grass patterns are carved on the lid surface. The pot, huge in size, neat in workmanship and shining with lustrous glaze, represents the productive level of lead-glazed pottery in the Han Dynasty.

Preserved in Shanxi Museum

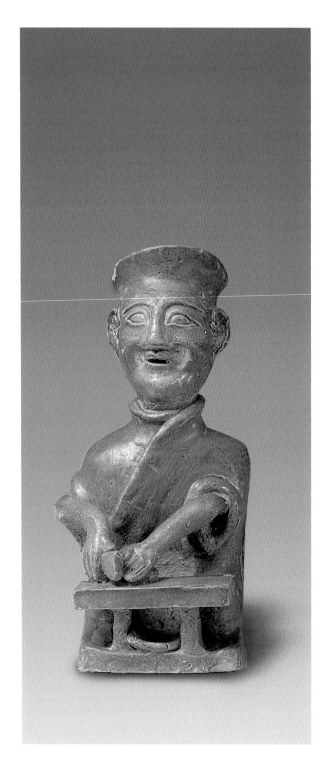

绿釉陶厨俑

东汉

釉陶质

高 29.8 厘米

Green-glazed Pottery Figurine of a Chef

Eastern Han Dynasty

Glazed Pottery

Height 29.8 cm

厨俑头戴帧，浓眉大眼，面露笑容，身着交领右衽袍，踞坐方案前，卷袖露臂，右手握刀，双手作切物状。案下置盆。全器满施绿釉。庖厨操作形态，生动逼真。与厨俑同墓出土的釉陶器，还有楼、井、磨、灶、壶、犬、鸡等，塑造精致。山东省高唐县东固河出土。

山东博物馆藏

The chef figurine, with a headscarf on his head, has bushy eyebrows, big eyes and a smiling face. Wearing a robe with a cross-collar and a right-lapel, he is kneeling in front of a squared chopping board, his sleeves rolled and his right hand holding a knife as if cutting something. There is a basin under the chopping board. The whole vessel is fully coated with green glaze. The chef's posture is vivid and true to life. Along with the chef figurine, some other glazed pottery objects unearthed from the same tomb, were all delicately designed, such as houses, wells, grinds, stoves, pots, dogs and chicken. This collection was excavated from Donggu River in Gaotang County, Shandong Province. Preserved in Shandong Museum

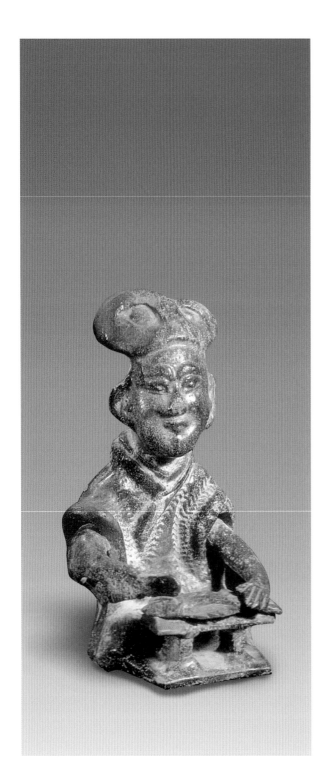

绿釉厨夫陶俑

东汉

泥质红陶

宽 11 厘米，高 21.5 厘米

Green-glazed Pottery Figurine of a Chef

Eastern Han Dynasty

Clay Red Pottery

Width 11 cm/ Height 21.5 cm

陶俑通体施绿釉，釉色绿中闪黄。头梳高髻，身着网纹短袖衫，束腰带，长裙，跽坐于案前。案上置鱼。俑左手执鱼尾，右手持刀作割鱼状。

河北博物馆藏

The whole vessel is fully coated with green glaze with a hint of yellow. The figurine, hair in an updo, wears a short-sleeved netlike shirt with a waistband and a long skirt, kneeling in front of a chopping board, where is laid a fish. She is holding the tail of the fish in her left hand and a knife in her right hand as if slicing the fish.

Preserved in Hebei Museum

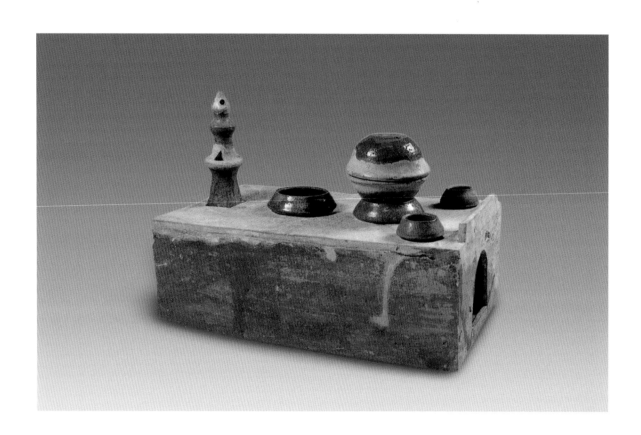

釉陶灶

东汉初

釉陶质

长 36.5 厘米，宽 22 厘米，高 27.5 厘米

Painted Pottery Stove

Early Eastern Han Dynasty

Glazed Pottery

Length 36.5 cm/ Width 22 cm/ Height 27.5 cm

此灶灶面上有两大两小4个火孔，小火孔上各放置1小釜，大火孔上的炊具有两种：1个单置1大釜；另一个则是1套甑釜组合炊具。这些器具约有不同分工：小釜用以温水，大釜用以煮羹制粥，甑釜组合是早期甗的替代品，是水烹汽蒸方式的具体体现。在同一个灶上同时烹饪不同的食品，一方面反映了汉代灶具的发达与先进，另一方面也说明汉代家庭人口众多。河南省济源市泗涧沟墓地出土。

河南省文物考古研究院藏

On the face of the stove are four fire holes, two small and two big. There is a small kettle placed on each of the small holes, while on the big holes are placed different kinds of cookers: a single big kettle and a cooking set including a rice steamer and a kettle. These cookwares function differently. The small kettle is for boiling water, and the big kettle for cooking porridge and soup. As the substitute for "Yan"(a combination of steamer and boiler) in the early times, the cooking set embodies the cooking style of boiling and steaming. The practice of cooking different food on different fire holes on the stove simultaneously not only indicates the advancement of the cooking utensils in Han Dynasty, but also shows the large size of the family then. This collection was unearthed from the Sijiangou tomb in Jiyuan City, Henan Province.

Preserved in Henan Provincial Institute of Cultural Heritage and Archaeology

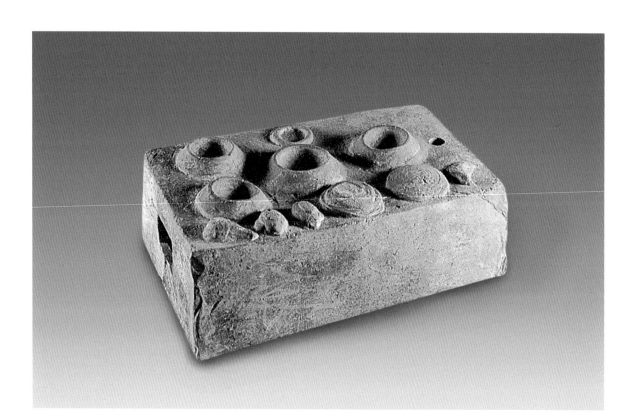

灰陶灶

东汉

灰陶质

长 23 厘米，宽 16 厘米，高 8 厘米

Grey Pottery Stove

Eastern Han Dynasty

Grey Pottery

Length 23 cm/ Width 16 cm/ Height 8 cm

平面长方形，横截面呈上小下大的梯形，一端有长方形的火门，灶面上有4个大小相若的火孔和1个圆形的烟道，烟囱已失。火孔上各放置有1个折腹的釜，均与灶连为一体。釜的两侧分别模印出1把勺、2只耳杯、1个盘、1个盆和1把炊帚，造型朴实无华，生活气息浓郁。河南省济源市轵国故城泗涧沟墓地出土。

河南省文物考古研究院藏

The plane surface of the stove is in the shape of a rectangle, and its transversal surface of a trapezoid with the lower part larger and the upper part smaller. On one side of the stove is a rectangular fire vent. On the cooking stove are four fire holes similar in size, and a round flue, with its chimney missing. On every fire hole is placed a kettle with a tapering ovoid body, which connects to the stove. On both sides of the kettles are moulded a spoon, two ear cups, a plate, a basin and a pot-scouring brush. The simple design of the stove reflects the rich flavor of genuine life. This collection was unearthed from a tomb at Sijiangou in the ancient city of Zhi State in Jiyuan City, Henan Province. Preserved in Henan Provincial Institute of Cultural Heritage and Archaeology

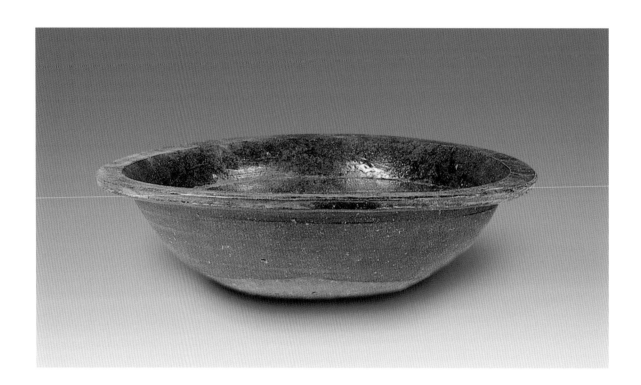

釉陶盆

东汉

釉陶质

口径 30.8 厘米，底径 15.5 厘米，高 8.1 厘米

Glazed Pottery Basin

Eastern Han Dynasty

Glazed Pottery

Mouth Diameter 30.8 cm/ Bottom Diameter 15.5 cm/ Height 8.1 cm

陶盆为方唇平折沿，曲腹大平底，底面内部下凹。内外均施彩釉，釉层不及底，所露胎骨为坚硬的褐红色。釉色分两种，盆内上部与沿面为豆绿色，余均呈棕红色，两种色釉相交处有一周弦纹，上下分界明显。釉层均匀而釉面亮泽，经揩拭光洁如新。河南省济源市轵国故城出土。

河南省文物考古研究院藏

This basin has an everted and flat mouth rim, a tapering ovoid body and a big flat bottom. with a concave interior. The exterior and interior of the basin are coated with coloured glazes, but the bottom is left unglazed, exposing its hard and brownish-red body. There are two glaze colours. The upper interior and the edge of the basin are coated with green glaze, while the remaining parts with brownish-red glaze. The interface of the two glazes is decorated with a ring of bowstring pattern, which clearly divide the upper and lower glazes. The glaze coating is even and lustrous. When cleaned with a cleaning rag, it looks like a newly-made basin. This collection was unearthed in an ancient city of the Zhi State in Jiyuan City, Henan Province.

Preserved in Henan Provincial Institute of Cultural Heritage and Archaeology

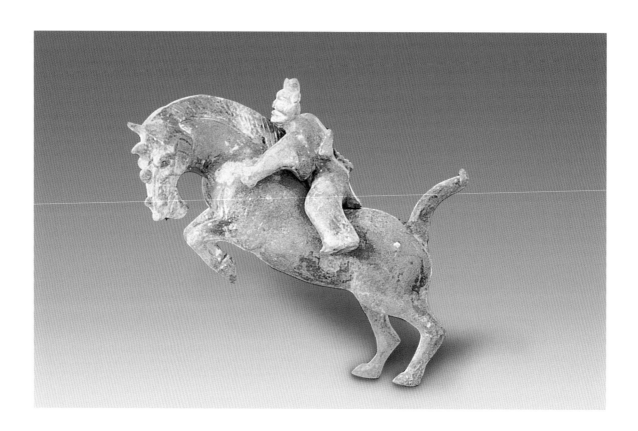

褐绿釉跃马陶俑

东汉

陶质

长 21 厘米

Brownish-green-glazed Figurine of Equestrian

Eastern Han Dynasty

Pottery

Length 21 cm

马的神态十足，作奔驰竞跃状，骑手匍匐于马背上。此俑展现了骑士于竞跑中的一个瞬间，动态感强烈。

徐氏艺术馆藏

The running horse was vividly designed as if it were racing with a rider sprawling on its back. This figurine portrays the dynamic moment of horse racing.

Preserved in The Tsui Museum of Art

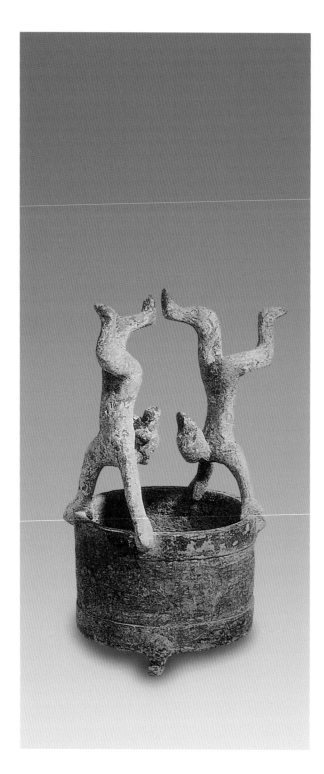

彩绘倒立技巧陶俑奁

东汉

泥质灰陶

高 19 厘米

Polychrome Pottery "Lian" (Dressing Case) with Handstand Acrobats

Eastern Han Dynasty

Clay Grey Pottery

Height 19 cm

在圆奁口沿上，相对倒立二俑，各以一腿相
对，另一腿自然向外屈伸。奁及二俑身上皆
涂朱彩。陶俑奁连型别致，二俑的技巧组合
巧妙，动作优美。

法国巴黎赛努奇博物馆

On the mouth rim of the circular dressing case
are two head-on handstand figurines with one
leg aiming at that of the other and the other leg
naturally flexing outwards. Thoroughly coated
with red colour, the pottery is uniquely shaped,
with the two figurines posing in a skillful and
elegant way.

Preserved in Musée Cernuschi，France

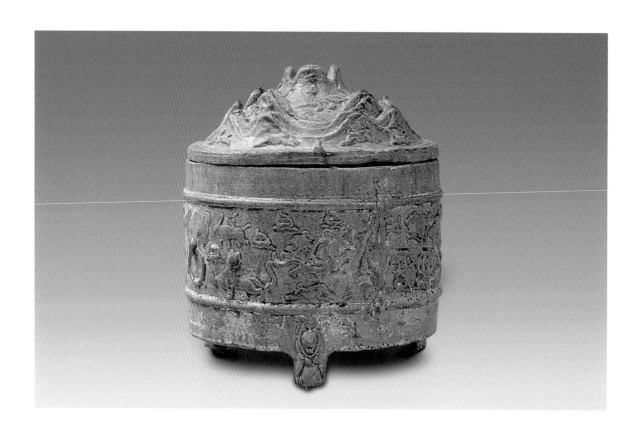

绿釉博山盖陶奁

东汉

陶质

口径 19 厘米，高 22.5 厘米

Green-glazed "Lian" (Dressing Case) with Boshan-style Lid

Eastern Han Dynasty

Pottery

Mouth Diameter 19 cm/ Height 22.5 cm

奁盖为博山式，盖上隆起塑成海上三山，有
珍禽瑞兽出没其间，盖边缘饰一周锯齿文。
奁身为筒式，平底，三熊足。腹体两端各饰
一周凸弦纹，周身饰山峰、街环铺首、羽人、
猛虎、兔子、奔鹿、猴、狮、人骑兽等纹饰，
均系模印而成。通体罩翠绿釉，晶亮莹润。

南京市博物馆藏

The dressing case comes with a Boshan-style lid on which are moulded the scene of three mountains in the ocean in relief with rare birds and auspicious beasts on them. The saw-toothed patterns are decorated on the edge of the lid. The case has a tubular body, a flat bottom and three bear feet. Both ends of the body are decorated with a tier of convex string patterns, while in between the two ends are stamped motifs including mountains, beast heads with a ring in the mouth, immortals capable of flying, fierce tigers, rabbits, running deers, monkeys, lions and people riding on beasts. The whole body of the case is covered with smooth and bright green glaze.

Preserved in Nanjing Museum

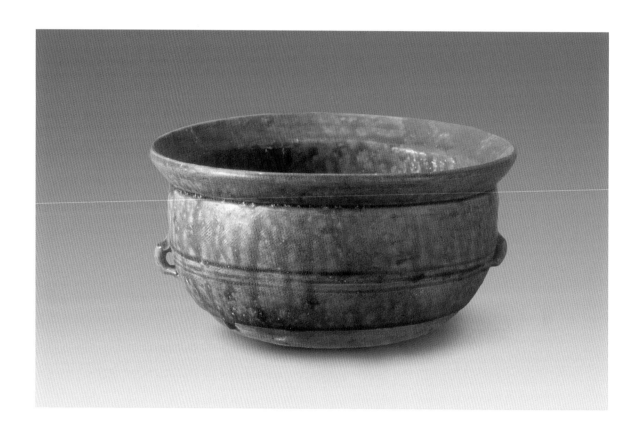

青瓷洗

东汉

瓷质

口径 25.7 厘米，底径 12.1 厘米，高 15.6 厘米

Celadon Washer

Eastern Han Dynasty

Porcelain

Mouth Diameter 25.7 cm/ Bottom Diameter 12.1 cm/ Height 15.6 cm

此器宽折沿，圆唇外翻，上腹直壁，下腹斜弧向下收成大平底，腹中部外壁饰三道弦纹，弦纹中间置对称桥形双耳。整器施青黄色釉，具有较强光泽，胎釉结合牢固，釉质晶莹呈半透明状，有冰裂纹。外壁施釉不及底，内壁有流釉痕迹。1991 年于邗江甘泉镇姚湾村吴庄出土。

扬州市邗江区文物管理委员会藏

This washer has a wide everted mouth rim and a round flared mouth, a straight upper belly and a lower belly tapering downward to the flat bottom. The exterior wall of the middle belly are decorated with three rings of string patterns, in between which symmetrically arranged a pair of bridge-shaped handles. The body is firmly coated with bright greenish-yellow glaze. The glaze with ice crackles is translucent and crystal-clear. The exterior wall of the washer is glazed except the bottom, and saggings can be found on the interior wall. The collection was excavated from Wu Manor of Yaowan Village, in Ganquan Town of Hanjiang Region, Jiangsu Province, in the year 1991.

Preserved in the Department of Cultural Relics Conservation, Hanjiang District, Yangzhou City

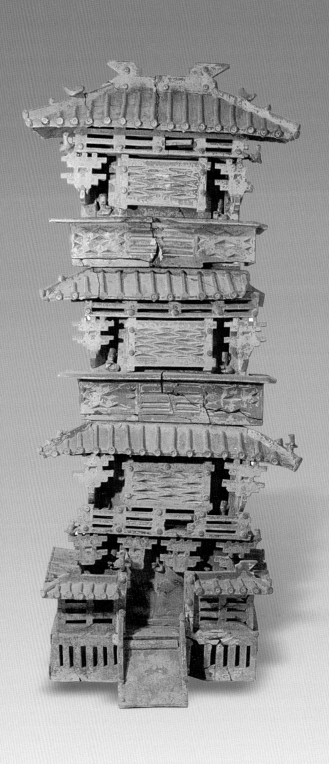

绿釉陶楼

东汉

釉陶质

通高 144 厘米，面阔 64 厘米，进深 36 厘米

泥质红陶，施绿釉。楼分四层，用两个圈座套叠。四阿式顶，有鸟形脊饰，各层有斗拱及廊檐，底座有台阶及立柱，柱上有鸟形饰。各层有长方形窗 35 个，窗口各有一人作探头招手状。陶楼层次较高，结构复杂，制作精细，为墓室明器。1978 年山东省宁津县大柳镇庞家寺出土。

宁津县图书馆藏

Green-glazed Pottery Tower

Eastern Han Dynasty

Glazed Pottery

Height 144 cm/ Width 64 cm/ Depth 36 cm

The clay red pottery is coated with green glaze. This four-storeyed tower has two telescopic seating, a hip roof with a bird pattern decorated on its ridges, corbel brackets and corridors on each floor, and a base with steps and pillars also decorated by bird patterns. On each floor are incised 35 rectangular windows. From each window can be seen a person sticking his head out and waving his hand. This high-rise building is a complex and exquisite burial object. It was unearthed in Pangjia Temple, Daliu Town, Ningjing County, Shandong Province, in the year 1978.

Preserved in Ningjin Library

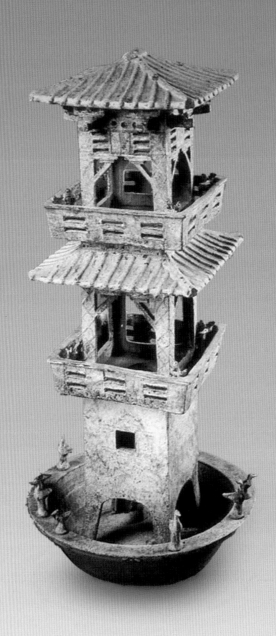

绿釉陶望楼

东汉

泥质红陶

通高 90.5 厘米

平底折沿圆池。通体饰绿釉。池沿立有数只家鸭。池中矗立四阿式三层楼阁。一层开一独窗。二层为四柱承托的楼阁，方形底座的四角，均有一位执弓守卫的护院武士，呈张弓欲射状。三层的构造同于二层，四角也各立有一执弓武士。

法国吉美国立亚洲艺术博物馆藏

Green-glazed Pottery Watch-tower

Eastern Han Dynasty

Clay Red Pottery

Height 90.5 cm

The object is fully coated with green glaze. The base of this watch-tower is a circular flat-bottomed pool with a flanged rim, around which stand several ducks. In the pool erects a three-storeyed pavilion with a hip roof. On the first floor, a window can be found. The second and third floor are designed similarly with four pillar supports and four court guards with bows and arrows in hand standing at the four corners, looking as if they were going to draw the bows to shoot.

Preserved in Musée National des Arts Asiatiques-Guimet, France

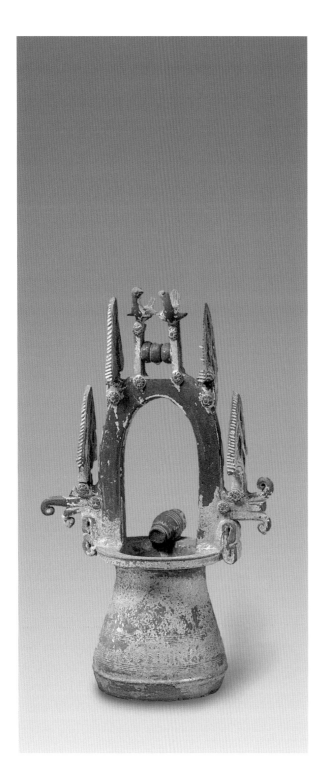

绿釉陶井

东汉

泥质红陶

底径 16 厘米，宽 30 厘米，通高 48 厘米

Green-glazed Pottery Well

Eastern Han Dynasty

Clay Red Pottery

Bottom Diameter 16 cm/ Width 30 cm/ Height 48 cm

红陶，施绿釉。井呈束腰筒状，平底，井口上竖拱形井亭，安有滑车及水桶，两侧饰有树叶，顶立二鸟，回眸相视，生活气息甚浓。庞家寺墓葬出土整套陶宅院、陶井建筑模型及大量生活器具，是汉代豪强地主庄园的缩影。1978年山东省宁津县大柳镇庞家寺出土。

宁津县图书馆藏

Coated with green glaze, this red pottery well has a waisted neck, a spraovading tubular body, and a flat bottom. On its mouth stands an arched pavilion equipped with a pulley and a bucket. Its two sides are decorated with leaf designs, with two birds standing on the top staring backward at each other. This image is vividly designed. As the miniature of the despotic landlord in the Han Dynasty, Pang Jia Temple Tombs is the birth place of a complete set of pottery messuage, models of pottery well and large numbers of household utensils. This well was unearthed from Pang Jia Temple in Daliu Town of Ningjin County, Shandong Province, in the year 1978.

Preserved in Ningjin Library

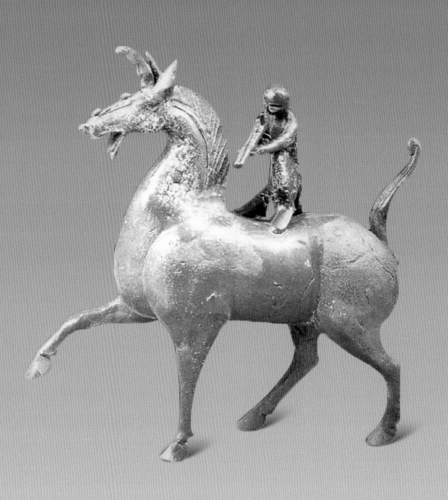

褐绿釉彩射俑

东汉

长 25 厘米

马神态生动，右足抬起，头部微弯向下，开口露齿呈嘶鸣状。骑俑右膝跪于马背上，手持弩机，正在瞄准行射。该俑充分展现了汉代骑马弩射的场景。

徐氏艺术馆藏

Brown Green Glazed Archer Warrior

Eastern Han Dynasty

Length 25cm

The horse is vividly molded. It lifts its right leg, lowers its head slightly and opens its mouth as if bellowing. The warrior kneels on the horse. He holds a crossbow and prepares to shoot. This fully reflects the situation of riding and shooting during Han Dynasty.

Preserved in The Tsui Museum of Art

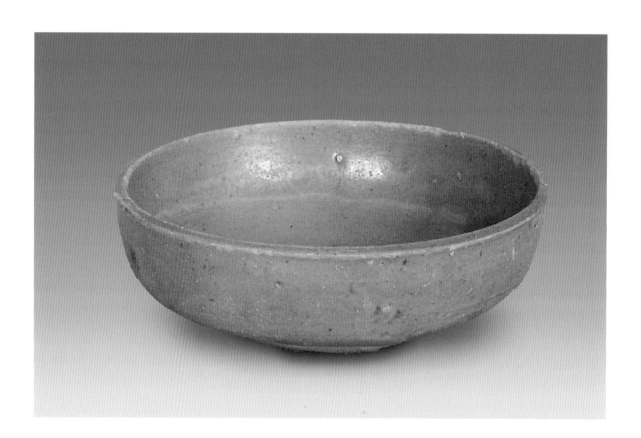

陶药洗

汉

陶质

口外径 12.7 厘米，高 4.5 厘米，壁厚 0.4 厘米

Pottery Medical Washer

Han Dynasty

Pottery

Outer Mouth Diameter 12.7 cm/ Height 4.5 cm/ Wall Thickness 0.4 cm

该藏品为圆碟形，由陶制成，施墨绿釉，平底直口，工艺粗糙，为医用药洗工具。保存基本完好。1955 年入藏。

中华医学会 / 上海中医药大学医史博物馆藏

This washer is in the shape of a round plate. Coated with blackish green glaze, the washer with a flat bottom and a straight mouth is rough in craftsmanship. It was used as a medical device for cleaning and disinfecting, and has been kept intact. The object was collected in the year 1955.

Preserved in Chinese Medical Association/ Museum of Chinese Medicine, Shanghai University of Traditional Chinese Medicine

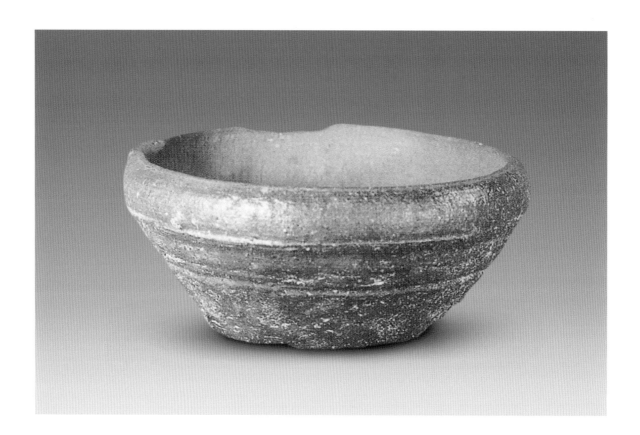

研钵

汉

陶质

口径 21 厘米，底径 11 厘米，高 8.5 厘米

Mortar

Han Dynasty

Pottery

Mouth Diameter 21 cm/ Bottom Diameter 11 cm/ Height 8.5 cm

该藏品厚重，胎体坚硬，可用于研磨药物。

上海中医药博物馆藏

This mortar is thick and heavy, with a hard body. It was used for porphyrizing traditional Chinese medicine.
Preserved in Shanghai Museum of Traditional Chinese Medicine

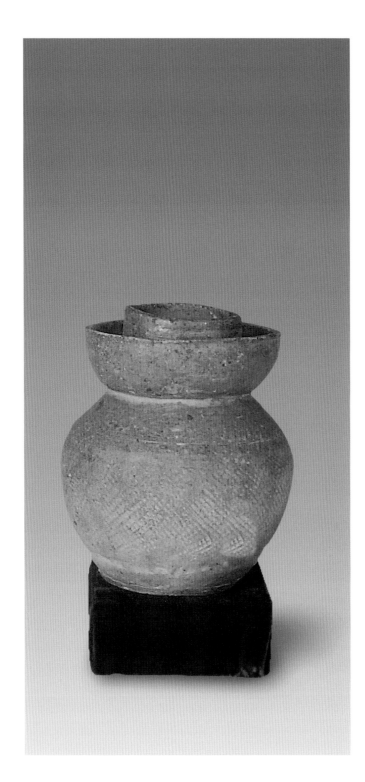

陶药壶

汉

陶质

口径 13.3 厘米，腹径 16.1 厘米，底径
9.7 厘米，通高 18.2 厘米

Pottery Medicine Pot

Han Dynasty

Pottery

Mouth Diameter 13.3 cm/ Belly Diameter
16.1 cm/ Bottom Diameter 9.7 cm/ Height
18.2 cm

该药壶为黄褐陶制成。施半面釉，平底直口双唇，缺盖，饰蓖点纹，壶身浅刻"丸"字，造型别致，工艺粗糙。盛药器具，保存基本完好。

中华医学会 / 上海中医药大学医史博物馆藏

This pot is made of ocher pottery. With half side glazed, the pot has a flat bottom, a straight mouth, and double lips with the lid missing. Adorned with castor spot patterns, the pot has a Chinese character "Wan" (pill) Lightly carved on its belly. The shape is exotic, though rough in craftsmanship. This pot is a medicine container and has been kept intact.

Preserved in Chinese Medical Association/ Museum of Chinese Medicine, Shanghai University of Traditional Chinese Medicine

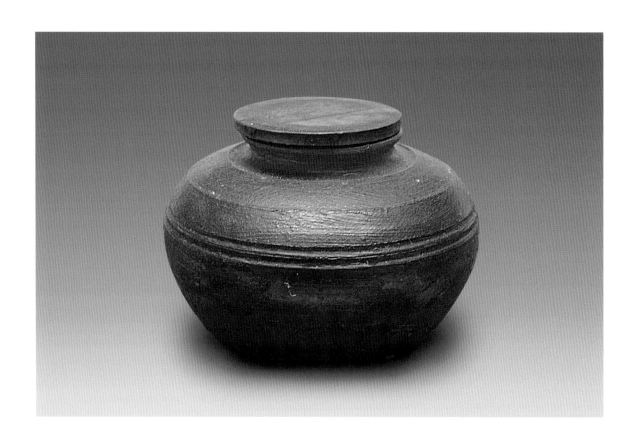

药罐

汉

陶质

口径 8 厘米，高 15 厘米

Pottery Medicine Jar

Han Dynasty

Pottery

Mouth Diameter 8 cm/ Height 15 cm

圆口，束颈，鼓腹，平底。腹中部有三道旋纹，圆饼形盖。器身髹红色漆。保存完好。成都市考古队征集。

成都中医药大学中医药传统文化博物馆藏

This jar is designed with a circular mouth, a contracted neck, a flat bottom and a swelling abdomen, in the middle of which are three bands of whorl patterns. With a round pie-shaped lid, the jar is coated with red lacquer and has been kept intact. It was collected by the archaeological team of Chengdu City, Sichuan Province.

Preserved in Museum of Traditional Chinese Medicine Culture, Chengdu University of Traditional Chinese Medicine

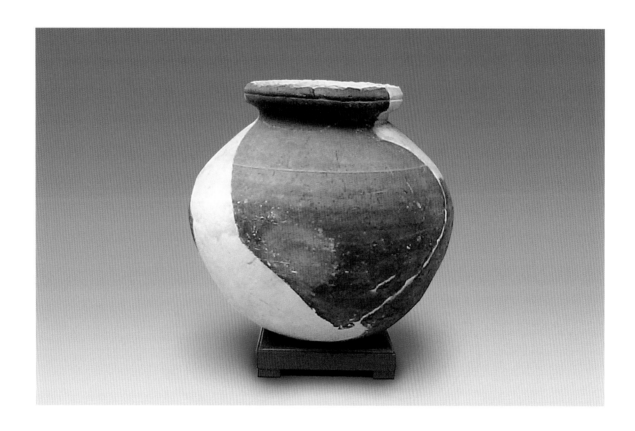

陶罐

汉

灰陶质

口外径 13.7 厘米，腹径 22.4 厘米，通高 23 厘米

Pottery Jar

Han Dynasty

Grey Pottery

Outer Mouth Diameter 13.7 cm/ Belly Diameter 22.4 cm/ Height 23 cm

该罐为碎陶片修复成型，表面有旋纹，尖底卷沿，无纹饰，制作精细，造型美观。为盛药器具。

上海中医药博物馆藏

The jar is restored and assembled from large original fragments. There are spiral patterns on the surface of the body. It has a pointed bottom and a rolled rim with no other decoration. The jar is exquisite in craftsmanship and attractive in appearance. It is a medicine storage container. Preserved in Shanghai Museum of Traditional Chinese Medicine

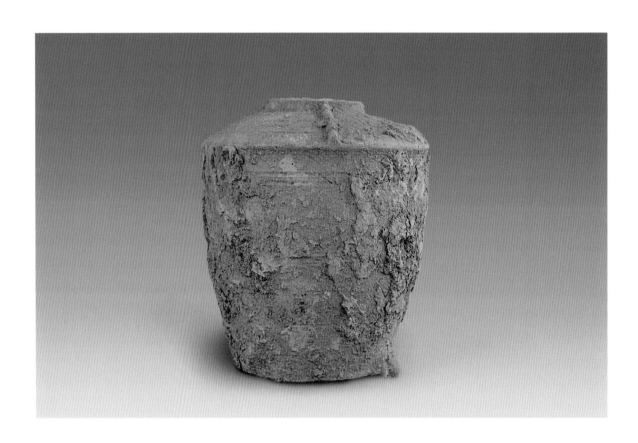

陶仓

汉

陶质

口径 10 厘米，底径 15 厘米，通高 25 厘米，重 2700 克

Pottery Granary

Han Dynasty

Pottery

Mouth Diameter 10 cm/ Bottom Diameter 15 cm/ Height 25 cm/ Weight 2,700 g

小口圆唇，折肩斜腹，三足，肩上有三凸棱。
一足有残。盛贮器。陕西省西安市长安区
征集。

陕西医史博物馆藏

This granary features a small mouth with a
circular rim, an angular shoulder, a sloping
abdomen, and three feet, one of which is cracked.
There are three raised ridges on the shoulder. The
object was used as a container. It was collected
from Chang'an District of Xi'an City, Shaanxi
Province.

Preserved in Shaanxi Museum of Medical History

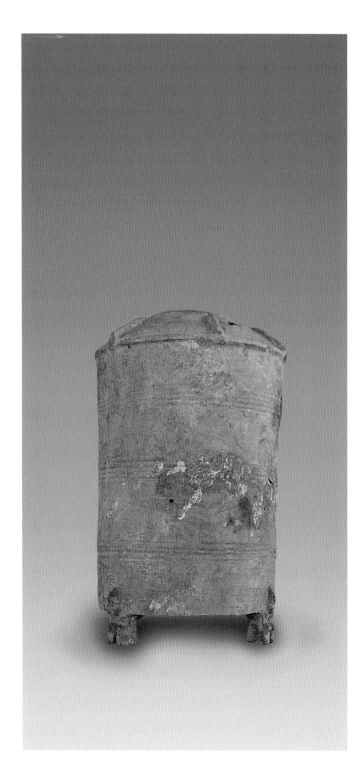

绿釉陶仓

汉

陶质

口径 9 厘米，底径 17.5 厘米，通高 31
厘米，重 3400 克

Green-glazed Pottery Granary

Han Dynasty

Pottery

Mouth Diameter 9 cm/ Bottom Diameter

17.5 cm/ Height 31 cm/ Weight 3,400 g

小口，圆唇，折肩直腹，三鼠足，肩上有六凸棱。一足残，肩有一小孔。盛贮器。陕西省西安市长安区征集。

陕西医史博物馆藏

This granary is designed with a small mouth, a circular rim, an angular shoulder, a straight abdomen, and three rat-paw-shaped feet, one of which is cracked. There are six raised ridges and a small hole on the shoulder. The object was utilized as a container. It was collected from Chang'an District of Xi'an City, Shaanxi Province.

Preserved in Shaanxi Museum of Medical History

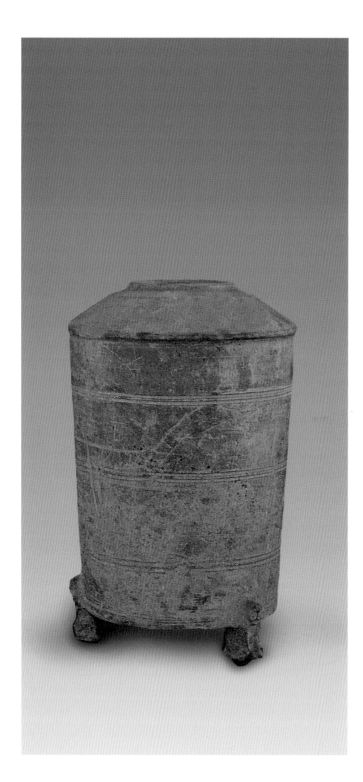

陶仓

汉

灰陶质

口径 7.5 厘米，底径 14.5 厘米，通高
26 厘米，重 1750 克

Pottery Granary

Han Dynasty

Grey Pottery

Mouth Diameter 7.5 cm/ Bottom Diameter
14.5 cm/ Height 26 cm/ Weight 1,750 g

小圆口，折肩，直腹，三足鼠足形，腹部
有三组弦纹。一足残损，余均完整。明器，
贮藏粮食。陕西省西安市长安区康申利上
交征集。

陕西医史博物馆藏

This granary has a small circular mouth, an
angular shoulder, a straight abdomen, and three
rat-paw-shaped feet. The abdomen is decorated
with three sets of raised horizontal lines. With
one of the feet cracked, the other parts of the
object remain intact. Used as a container for
storing grain, the granary is a burial object. It
was donated by Kang Shenli from Chang'an
District, Xian'City, Shaanxi Province.
Preserved in Shaanxi Museum of Medical History

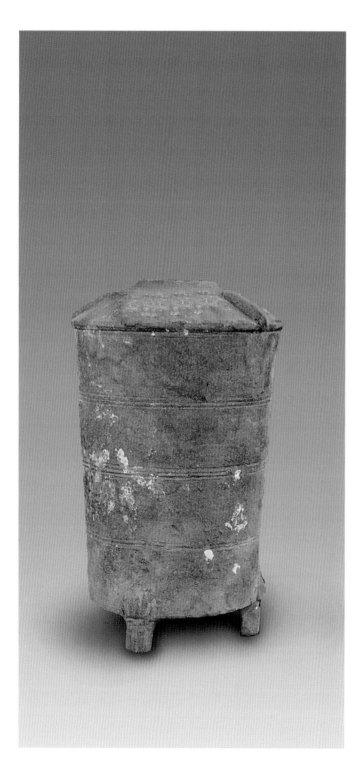

陶仓

汉

带釉陶质

口径 7.5 厘米，底径 15.8 厘米，通高
33 厘米，重 3850 克

Pottery Granary

Han Dynasty

Glazed Pottery

Mouth Diameter 7.5 cm/ Bottom Diameter

15.8 cm/ Height 33 cm/ Weight 3,850 g

小圆口，折肩，直斜腹，三鼠足，腹部有三
周弦纹饰，肩部有五凸棱。完整无损。明器，
粮仓。陕西省西安市长安区康申利上交征集。

陕西医史博物馆藏

This granary features a small circular mouth,
an angular shoulder with five raised ridges, a
vertical sloping abdomen, and three rat-paw-
shaped feet. The abdomen is decorated with
three bands of raised horizontal lines. The
granary is a burial object and has been kept
intact. It was donated by Kang Shenli from
Chang'an District, Xian'City, Shaanxi Province.
Preserved in Shaanxi Museum of Medical History

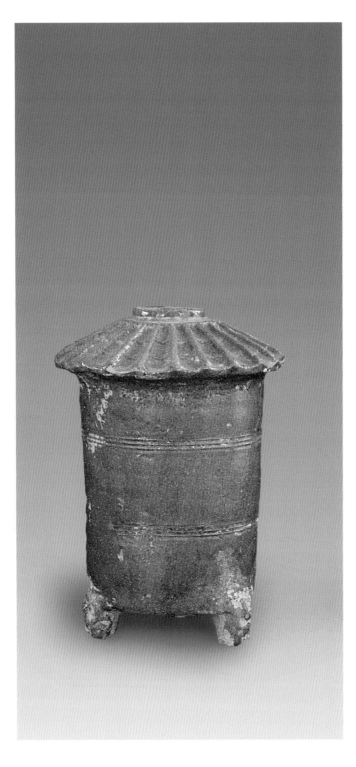

陶仓

汉

釉陶质

口径 5.5 厘米，底径 13 厘米，通高 44 厘米，重 1800 克

Pottery Granary

Han Dynasty

Glazed Pottery

Mouth Diameter 5.5 cm/ Bottom Diameter

13 cm/ Height 44 cm/ Weight 1,800 g

小圆口，肩围伞形，直腹，三竖足，腹部有两周弦纹。完整无损。明器，贮藏器具。陕西省咸阳市窑店胡春芳上交征集。

陕西医史博物馆藏

This granary has a small circular mouth, an umbrella-shaped shoulder, a straight abdomen and three vertical feet. The abdomen is decorated with two bands of raised horizontal lines. Utilized as a container for storage, this funeral object has been kept intact. It was donated by Hu Chunfang from Yaodian County, Xianyang City, Shaanxi Province.

Preserved in Shaanxi Museum of Medical History

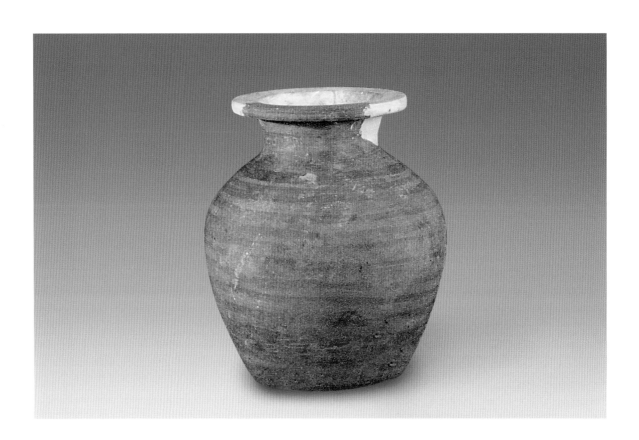

陶瓶

汉

陶质

口径 12 厘米，底径 11 厘米，通高 19 厘米，1400 克

Pottery Vase

Han Dynasty

Pottery

Mouth Diameter 12 cm/ Bottom Diameter 11 cm/ Height 19 cm/ Weight 1,400 g

盘口，溜肩，圆腹，平底，腹有环状纹。口沿有修补。盛贮器。

陕西医史博物馆藏

This pottery vase has a dish-shaped mouth, a sloping shoulder, a round abdomen decorated with ring patterns and a flat bottom. The mouth rim is repaired. The object was used as a storage container.

Preserved in Shaanxi Museum of Medical History

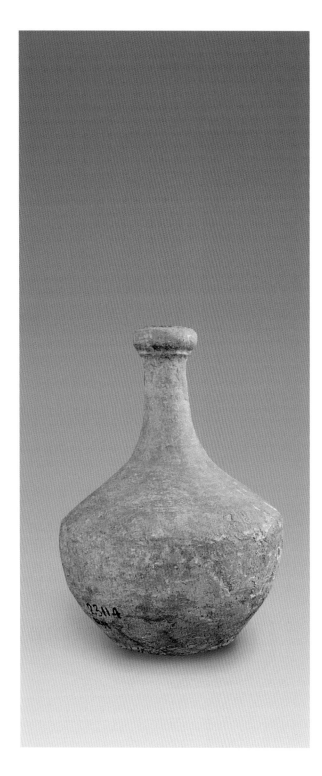

蒜头瓶

汉

陶质

口径 5.5 厘米，底径 11 厘米，通高 27 厘米，
重 1400 克

Garlic-head Vase

Han Dynasty

Pottery

Mouth Diameter 5.5 cm/ Bottom Diameter 11 cm/

Height 27 cm/ Weight 1,400 g

蒜头口，长细颈，折肩圆腹，平底。完整无损。
盛储器。陕西省西安市南郊边家村征集。

陕西医史博物馆藏

The vase has a mouth in the shape of garlic
head, a long and thin neck, an angular shoulder,
a swelling belly and a flat bottom. It was
utilized as a storage container and has been kept
intact. The object was collected from Bianjia
village, southern suburbs of Xi'an City, Shaanxi
Province.

Preserved in Shaanxi Museum of Medical History

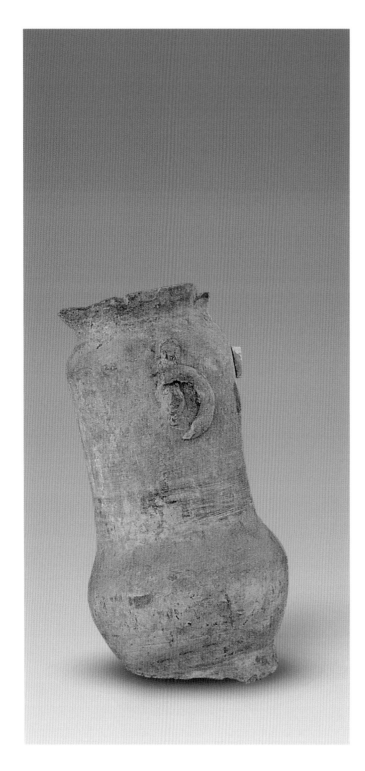

假双耳陶瓶

汉

陶质

口径13厘米，底径13厘米，通高30厘米，

重1550克

Pottery Vase with Two Decorating
Ears

Han Dynasty

Pottery

Mouth Diameter 13 cm/ Bottom Diameter

13 cm/ Height 30 cm/ Weight 1,550 g

侈口，颈长较粗，圆腹，圈足，有浮雕，双耳。
口沿底沿残。盛贮器。陕西省西安市半坡村
出土。

陕西医史博物馆藏

This vase, with relief carvings on the surface,
features a flared mouth, a long and relatively
thick neck, a swelling abdomen, a ring foot
and two ears. The rims of both the mouth and
bottom are cracked. It was utilized as a storage
container, and excavated from Banpo Village of
Xi'an city, Shaanxi Province.

Preserved in Shaanxi Museum of Medical History

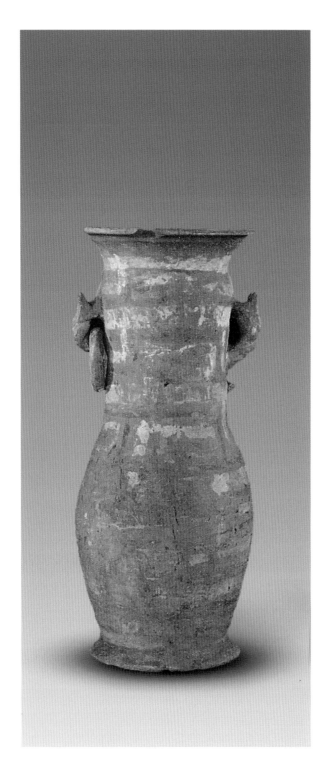

双耳彩绘陶瓶

汉

陶质

口径 14 厘米，底径 12 厘米，通高 33 厘米，
重 1600 克

Two-eared Painted Pottery Vase

Han Dynasty

Pottery

Mouth Diameter 14 cm/ Bottom Diameter 12 cm/

Height 33 cm/ Weight 1,600 g

盘口，长圆腹，浅喇叭底座，颈长较粗，颈
部兽头双耳，通体红白色彩绘。口沿、底沿
稍残。盛贮器。陕西省西安市半坡村出土。

陕西医史博物馆藏

This painted vase has a dish-shaped mouth, a
long and round abdomen, a shallow trumpet-
shaped base, and a long and relatively thick
neck. Two animal-head-shaped ears are
attached to the sides of the neck. The entire
vase is painted red and white. The rims of the
mouth and the bottom are slightly cracked. The
vase was utilized as a storage container and
unearthed from Banpo Village of Xi'an City,
Shaanxi Province.

Preserved in Shaanxi Museum of Medical History

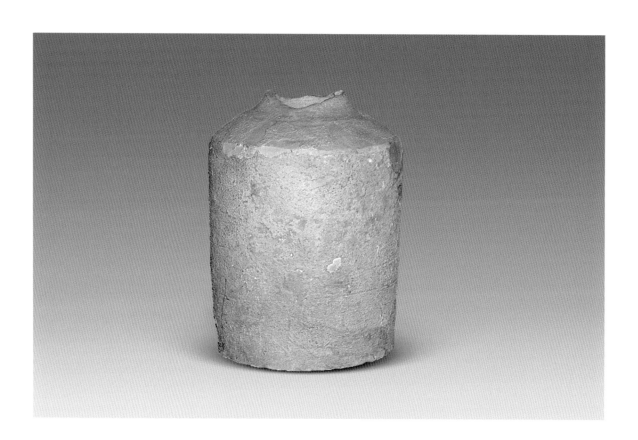

陶瓶

汉

陶质

口径 2.7 厘米，底径 10 厘米，高 14.2 厘米，重 700 克

Pottery Vase

Han Dynasty

Pottery

Mouth Diameter 2.7 cm/ Bottom Diameter 10 cm/ Height 14.2 cm/ Weight 700 g

斜肩，直腹，平底，素面，灰陶。口残。生
活器具。陕西省澄城县征集。

陕西医史博物馆藏

With the mouth cracked, this unglazed grey
pottery vase has an oblique shoulder, a straight
abdomen and a flat bottom. The vase served
as a household ware, and was collected from
Chengcheng County, Shaanxi Province.

Preserved in Shaanxi Museum of Medical History

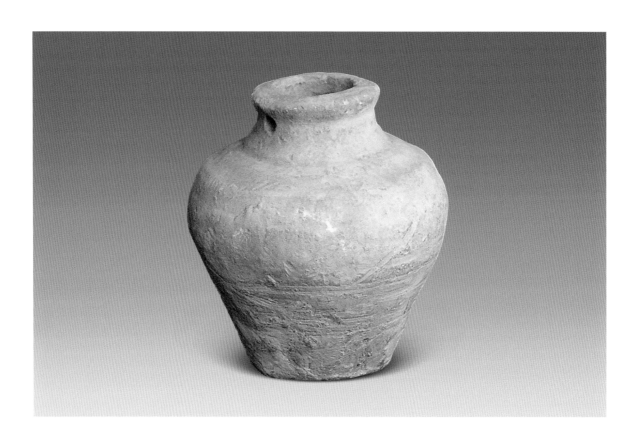

陶瓶

汉

陶质

口径 4 厘米，底径 4.5 厘米，高 9.4 厘米，重 300 克

Pottery Vase

Han Dynasty

Pottery

Mouth Diameter 4cm/ Bottom Diameter 4.5/Height 9.4cm/ Weight 300g

平口沿，短颈，斜肩，斜腹，平底，颈部有
两对称小孔，素面。灰陶。完整无损。生活
用器。陕西省澄城县征集。

陕西医史博物馆藏

This unglazed grey pottery vase features a
flat mouth rim, a short neck, a slant shoulder,
an oblique belly, and a flat bottom. Two
symmetrical holes can be found on the neck.
This well-kept vase served as a household ware,
and was collected from Chengcheng County,
Shaanxi Province.

Preserved in Shaanxi Museum of Medical History

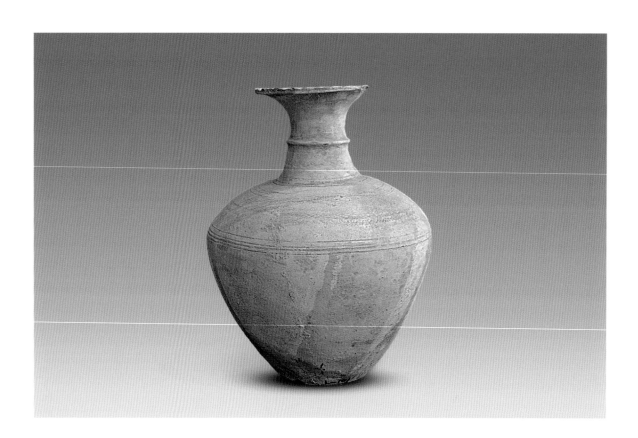

陶瓶

汉

陶质

口径 12.2 厘米，底径 9.6 厘米，高 30 厘米，重 2100 克

Pottery Vase

Han Dynasty

Pottery

Mouth Diameter 12.2 cm/ Bottom Diameter 9.6 cm/ Height 30 cm/ Weight 2,100 g

喇叭口，长颈，圆肩，斜腹，平底，灰陶，肩部数道弦纹，并饰有链条纹。口沿残。盛贮器。陕西省澄城县征集。

陕西医史博物馆藏

This grey pottery vase features a trumpet-shaped mouth, a long neck, a rounded shoulder, an oblique abdomen, and a flat bottom. The shoulder is adorned with several bands of raised horizontal lines and chain patterns. Its mouth rim is cracked. The vase served as a storage container and was collected from Chengcheng County, Shaanxi Province.

Preserved in Shaanxi Museum of Medical History

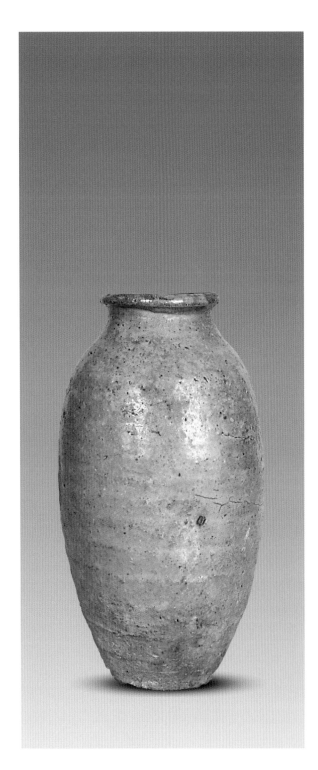

陶水瓶

汉

陶质

腹围 44.7 厘米，通高 26 厘米

Pottery Water Vase

Han Dynasty

Pottery

Abdominal Perimeter 44.7 cm/ Height 26 cm

该瓶为圆筒形，细沙灰白陶质，通身施乳白釉，平底，底面无釉无款识，烧制火候较高，表面粗糙。保存基本完好，口沿有残。为盛水器具。1960 年入藏。

中华医学会 / 上海中医药大学医史博物馆藏

This cylindrical vase is made of greyish white pottery mixed with fine sand grains. The vase is coated with opaline glaze, except the unglazed flat bottom which has no inscriptions. Fired at a relatively high temperature, it is rough on the outer surface. The water vase was used as a water container, and remains intact except for very small cracks on the rim. It was collected in the year 1960.

Preserved in Chinese Medical Association/ Museum of Chinese Medicine, Shanghai University of Traditional Chinese Medicine

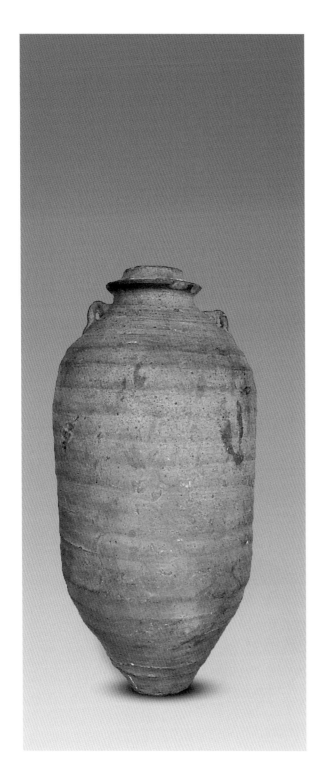

陶水瓶

汉

陶质

腹围 50.8 厘米，通高 32.5 厘米

Pottery Water Vase

Han Dynasty

Pottery

Abdominal Perimeter 50.8 cm/ Height 32.5 cm

该瓶为锥形瓶，黑灰色夹沙粗陶，烧制火候较高，表面粗糙，饰旋纹，平底，肩部有两系，是我馆仅藏不多的汉代陶瓷器之一。保存基本完好，口沿有残。为盛水器具。1960年入藏。

中华医学会／上海中医药大学医史博物馆藏

This cone-shaped vase is made of crude blackish-grey pottery with sand inclusion. Fired at a high temperature, the vase has a rough surface decorated with spiral patterns, a flat bottom and a shoulder with two rings. The vase is one of the few pottery wares of the Han Dynasty collected in the museum. The object, used as a water container, remains intact except for very small cracks on the rim. It was collected in the year 1960.

Preserved in Chinese Medical Association/ Museum of Chinese Medicine, Shanghai University of Traditional Chinese Medicine

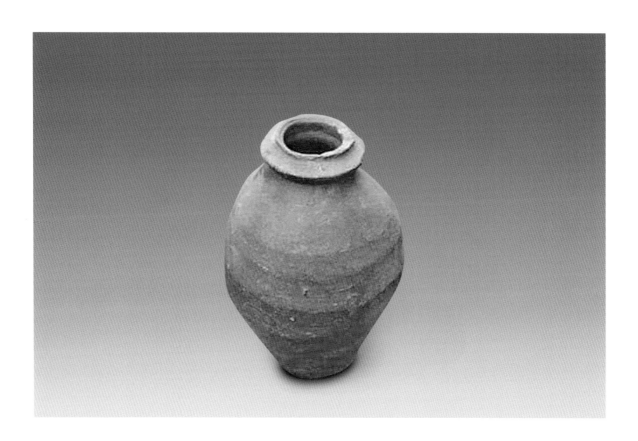

军持

汉

陶质

口外径 3 厘米，底径 5 厘米，腹径 10.4 厘米，腹深 14.3 厘米，通高 15 厘米，重 400 克

Kendis

Han Dynasty

Pottery

Outer Mouth Diameter 3 cm/ Bottom Diameter 5 cm/ Belly Diameter 10.4 cm/ Belly depth 14.3 cm/ Height 15 cm/ Weight 400 g

平口，鼓腹，腹深，腹下部内敛，平底。军持
一词来源于印度梵语，佛教僧侣饮水、洗手
等的容器，此物原题军持待考。

广东中医药博物馆藏

This kendis has a flat mouth, a deep swelling abdomen with the lower part narrowing down to a flat bottom. The word "kendis", which originated from Sanskrit (classical language of Indian), refers to a vessel used for drinking or washing hands by Buddhist monks. The original name of this object remains to be verified.

Preserved in Guangdong Chinese Medicine Museum

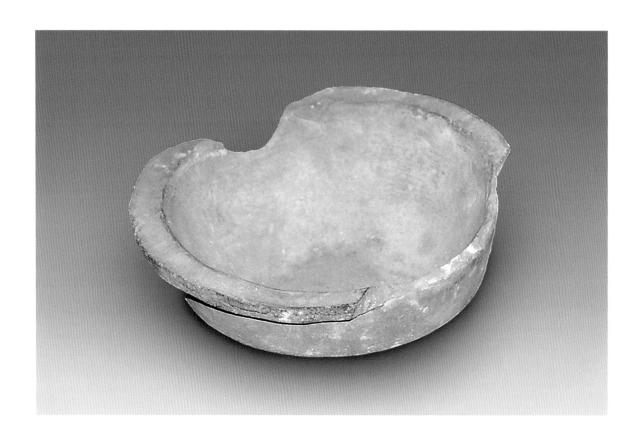

陶罐

汉

陶质

口径 9 厘米，底径 3.5 厘米，高 3.5 厘米，重 100 克

Pottery Jar

Han Dynasty

Pottery

Mouth Diameter 9 cm/ Bottom Diameter 3.5 cm/ Height 3.5 cm/ Weight 100 g

平口沿，折腹，平底，灰陶。口残。炊器。
陕西省澄城县征集。

陕西医史博物馆藏

This grey pottery jar is designed with a flat
mouth rim, an angular abdomen and a flat
bottom. The mouth rim is cracked. The jar
served as a cooking vessel, and was collected
from Chengcheng County, Shaanxi Province.

Preserved in Shaanxi Museum of Medical History

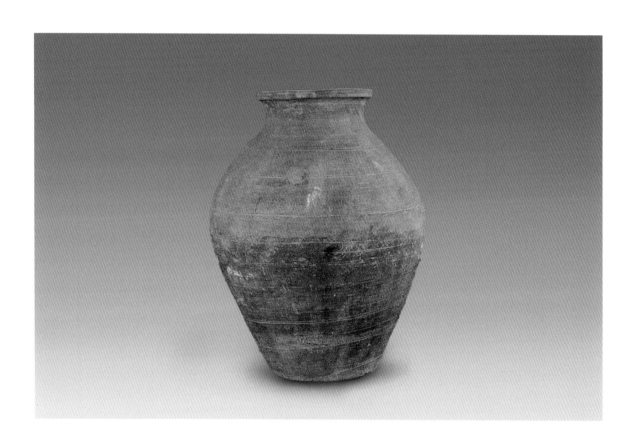

陶罐

汉

陶质

口径 13 厘米，通高 30.5 厘米，底径 12.4 厘米，重 3200 克

Pottery Jar

Han Dynasty

Pottery

Mouth Diameter 13 cm/ Height 30.5 cm/ Bottom Diameter 12.4 cm/ Weight 3,200 g

厚唇，鼓腹，平底，上腹有三道弦纹。完整无损。

盛贮器。陕西省西安市长安区康申利上交征集。

陕西医史博物馆藏

This pottery jar features a thick rim, a bulging body and a flat bottom. There are three bands of raised horizontal lines on the upper part of abdomen. The jar served as a storage container and has been kept intact. It was donated by Kang Shenli from Chang'an District, Xi'an City Shaanxi Province.

Preserved in Shaanxi Museum of Medical History

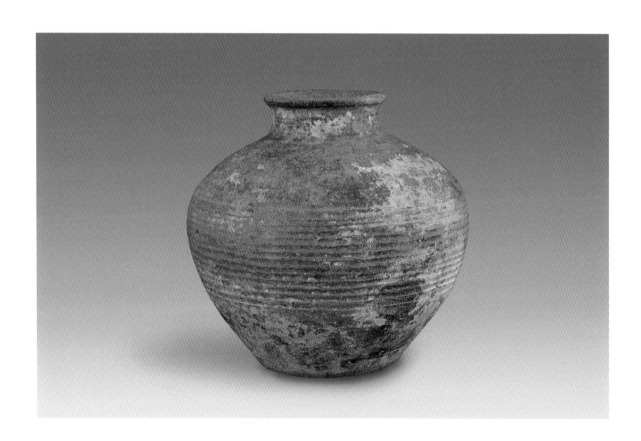

陶罐

汉

陶质

口径 9.6 厘米，底径 10.4 厘米，通高 20.1 厘米，重 1600 克

Pottery Jar

Han Dynasty

Pottery

Mouth Diameter 9.6 cm/ Bottom Diameter 10.4 cm/ Height 20.1 cm/ Weight 1,600 g

圆唇口，圆腹，平底，腹为粗弦纹饰。完整
无损。容器。陕西省澄城县征集。

陕西医史博物馆藏

This pottery jar has a circular-rimmed mouth, a
globular body and a flat bottom. The abdomen
is decorated with thick raised horizontal lines. It
served as a container and has been kept intact.
The jar was collected from Chengcheng County,
Shaanxi Province.

Preserved in Shaanxi Museum of Medical History

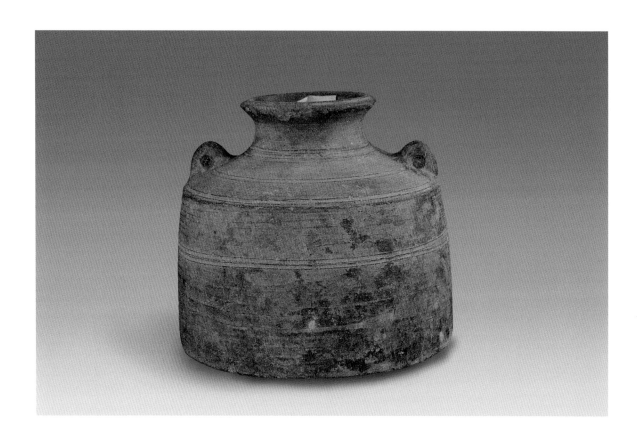

陶罐

汉

陶质

口径 11.6 厘米，底径 23.7 厘米，通高 20 厘米，重 3100 克

Pottery Jar

Han Dynasty

Pottery

Mouth Diameter 11.6 cm/ Bottom Diameter 23.7 cm/ Height 20 cm/ Weight 3,100 g

侈口，平肩，肩上有二耳，直腹平底。完整
无损。容器。陕西省澄城县征集。

陕西医史博物馆藏

This jar has a flared mouth, a flat shoulder with
two ears attached, a straight abdomen and a
flat bottom. It served as a container and has
been kept intact. The jar was collected from
Chengcheng County, Shaanxi Province.

Preserved in Shaanxi Museum of Medical History

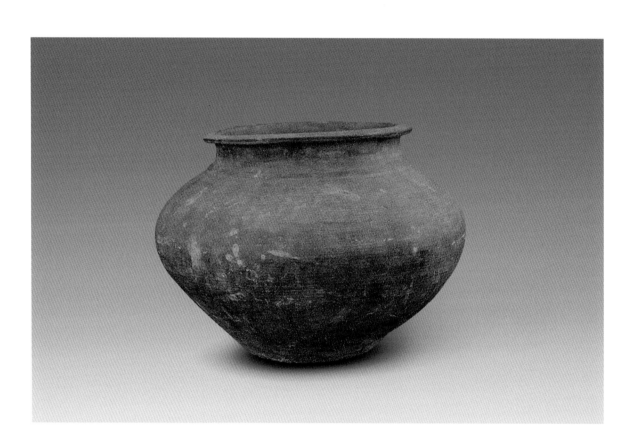

陶罐

汉

陶质

口径 17.8 厘米，底径 11 厘米，通高 17.8 厘米，重 2000 克

圆唇口，鼓腹，平底。完整无损。容器。陕西省澄城县征集。

陕西医史博物馆藏

Pottery Jar

Han Dynasty

Pottery

Mouth Diameter 17.8 cm/ Bottom Diameter 11 cm/ Height 17.8 cm/ Weight 2,000 g

This pottery jar has a circular-rimmed mouth, a globular body and a flat bottom. It served as a container and has been kept intact. The jar was collected from Chengcheng County, Shaanxi Province.

Preserved in Shaanxi Museum of Medical History

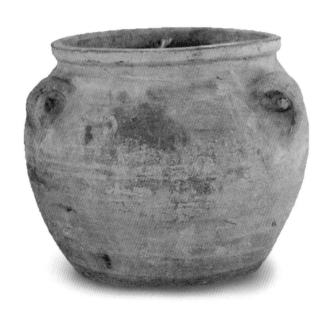

四耳陶罐

汉

陶质

口径 18 厘米，底径 16 厘米，通高 19 厘米，
重 1700 克

敞口，圆腹，平底，肩上有四耳。口沿处有一
裂纹。容器。陕西省澄城县征集。

陕西医史博物馆藏

Pottery Jar with Four Ears

Han Dynasty

Pottery

Mouth Diameter 18 cm/ Bottom Diameter 16 cm/
Height 19 cm/ Weight 1,700 g

This pottery jar has a flared mouth, a round belly, a
flat bottom and a shoulder with four ears attached.
This storage utensil with a crack on the mouth rim was
collected from Chengcheng County, Shaanxi Province.
Preserved in Shaanxi Museum of Medical History

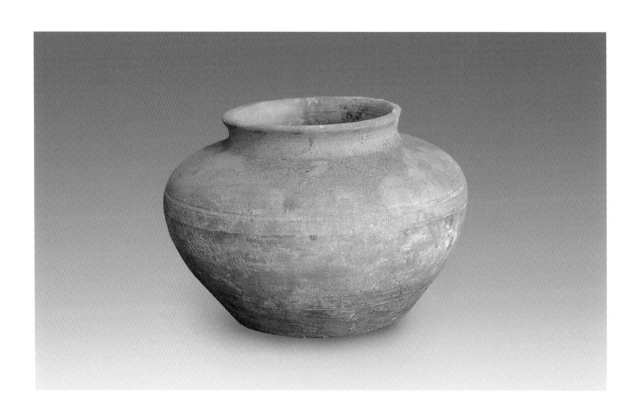

陶罐

汉

陶质

口径 10.6 厘米，底径 10.5 厘米，高 12 厘米，重 950 克

Pottery Jar

Han Dynasty

Pottery

Mouth Diameter 10.6 cm/ Bottom Diameter 10.5 cm/ Height 12 cm/ Weight 950 g

唇口，圆肩，斜腹，平底，肩部有一道弦纹，灰陶，素面。口沿残。生活器具。陕西省澄城县征集。

陕西医史博物馆藏

This pottery jar features a lip-shaped mouth, a round shoulder, a tapering ovoid body, and a flat bottom. The shoulder is decorated with a band of raised horizontal line. The plain jar, made of grey pottery, served as a storage utensil, with the mouth rim cracked. It was collected from Chengcheng County, Shaanxi Province.

Preserved in Shaanxi Museum of Medical History

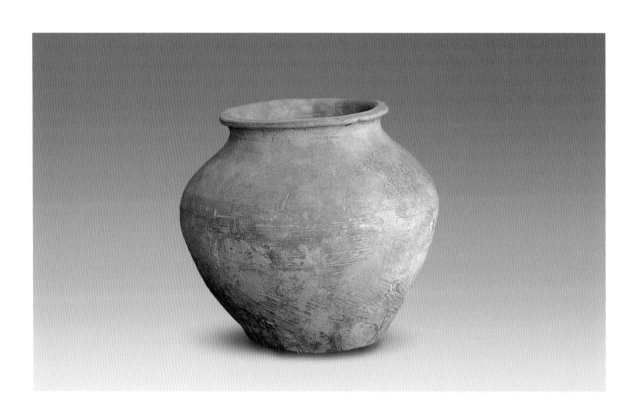

陶罐

汉

陶质

口径 14.8 厘米，底径 13.3 厘米，高 20.2 厘米，重 2600 克

Pottery Jar

Han Dynasty

Pottery

Mouth Diameter 14.8 cm/ Bottom Diameter 13.3 cm/ Height 20.2 cm/ Weight 2,600 g

圆唇，溜肩，斜腹，平底，灰陶，素面。完整
无损。盛贮器。陕西省澄城县征集。

陕西医史博物馆藏

The pottery jar is designed with a round rim, a
sloping shoulder, a tapering ovoid body, and a
flat bottom. This plain jar, made of grey pottery,
served as a storage utensil which remains intact.
It was collected from Chengcheng County,
Shaanxi Province.

Preserved in Shaanxi Museum of Medical History

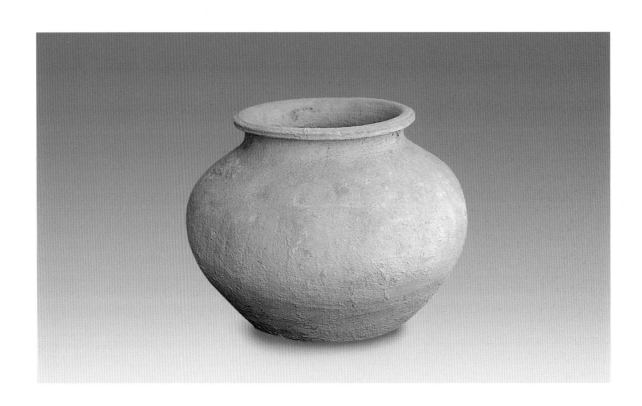

陶罐

汉

陶质

口径 13.8 厘米，底径 12.2 厘米，高 16 厘米，重 1600 克

圆唇，斜肩，圆腹，平底，素面，灰陶。完整无损。盛贮器。陕西省澄城县征集。

陕西医史博物馆藏

Pottery Jar

Han Dynasty

Pottery

Mouth Diameter 13.8 cm/ Bottom Diameter 12.2 cm/ Height 16cm/ Weight 1,600 g

This grey pottery jar, with no decoration, features a round rim, a sloping shoulder, a globular body, and a flat bottom. This storage utensil was collected from Chengcheng County, Shaanxi Province, and remains intact.

Preserved in Shaanxi Museum of Medical History

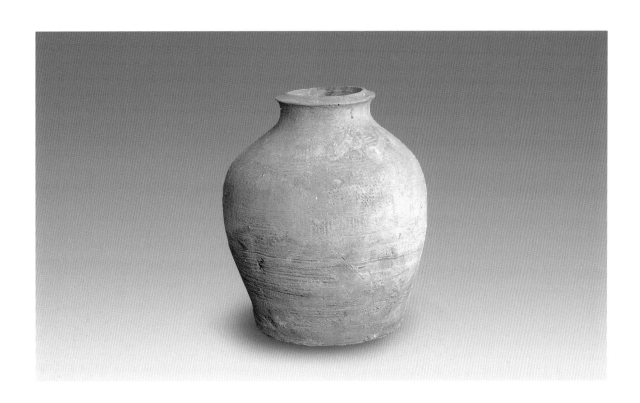

陶罐

汉

陶质

口径 7 厘米，底径 10.4 厘米，高 16.8 厘米，重 1300 克

平口沿，溜肩，直斜腹，平底，灰陶，素面。完整无损。盛贮器。陕西省澄城县征集。

陕西医史博物馆藏

Pottery Jar

Han Dynasty

Pottery

Mouth Diameter 7 cm/ Bottom Diameter 10.4 cm/ Height 16.8 cm/ Weight 1,300 g

This plain grey pottery jar features a flat mouth rim, a sloping shoulder, a slightly tapering body, and a flat bottom. This storage utensil was collected from Chengcheng County, Shaanxi Province, and remains intact.

Preserved in Shaanxi Museum of Medical History

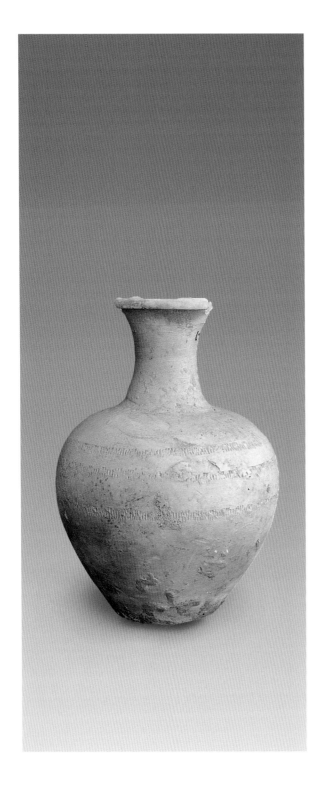

陶瓶

汉

陶质

口径 4.7 厘米，底径 7.3 厘米，高 22 厘米，重 1000 克

Pottery Vase

Han Dynasty

Pottery

Mouth Diameter 4.7 cm/ Bottom Diameter 7.3 cm/ Height 22 cm/ Weight 1,000 g

喇叭口，长颈，圆肩，圆腹，平底，腹部三
道指甲纹,灰陶。肩、腹各有一洞,口沿3/4残。
盛贮器。陕西省澄城县征集。

陕西医史博物馆藏

This grey pottery jar features a mouth in the
shape of a trumpet, a long neck, a rounded
shoulder, a round belly surrounded with three
bands of fingernail patterns, and a flat bottom.
There is a hole on the shoulder and another
on the belly. Three fourths of the mouth rim is
cracked. This storage utensil was collected from
Chengcheng County, Shaanxi Province.
Preserved in Shaanxi Museum of Medical History

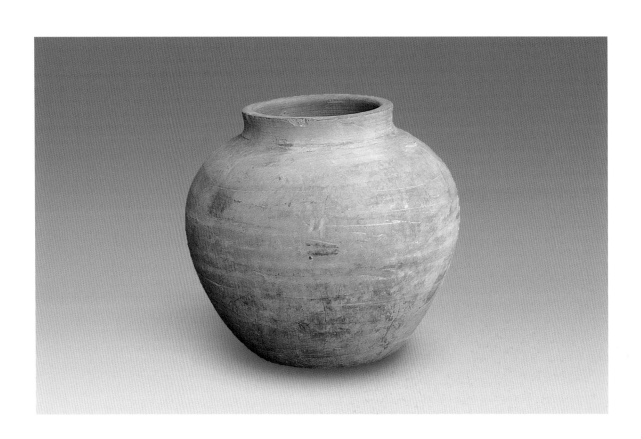

陶罐

汉

陶质

口径 9 厘米，底径 9 厘米，高 14.3 厘米，重 650 克

直口，圆腹，平底，灰陶，素面。完整无损。盛贮器。陕西省澄城县征集。

陕西医史博物馆藏

Pottery Jar

Han Dynasty

Pottery

Mouth Diameter 9 cm/ Bottom Diameter 9 cm/ Height 14.3 cm/ Weight 650 g

This unglazed pottery jar features a straight mouth, a globular body, and a flat bottom. This storage utensil remains intact and was collected from Chengcheng County, Shaanxi Province.

Preserved in Shaanxi Museum of Medical History

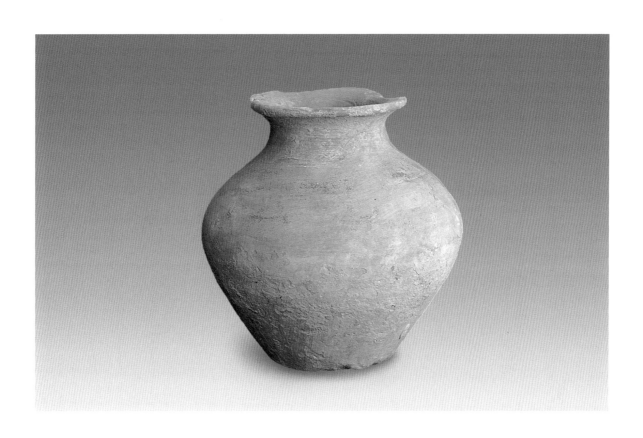

陶罐

汉

陶质

口径 11 厘米，底径 9.5 厘米，高 8.5 厘米，重
1500 克

小喇叭口，溜肩，折腹，平底，灰陶，素面。口
沿残。盛贮器。陕西省澄城县征集。

陕西医史博物馆藏

Pottery Jar

Han Dynasty

Pottery

Mouth Diameter 11 cm/ Bottom Diameter 9.5 cm/
Height 8.5 cm/ Weight 1,500 g

This unglazed grey pottery jar has a small trumpet-
shaped mouth, a sloping shoulder, an angular belly,
and a flat bottom. The mouth aim is cracked. This
object served as a storage utensil, and was collected
from Chengcheng County, Shaanxi Province.

Preserved in Shaanxi Museum of Medical History

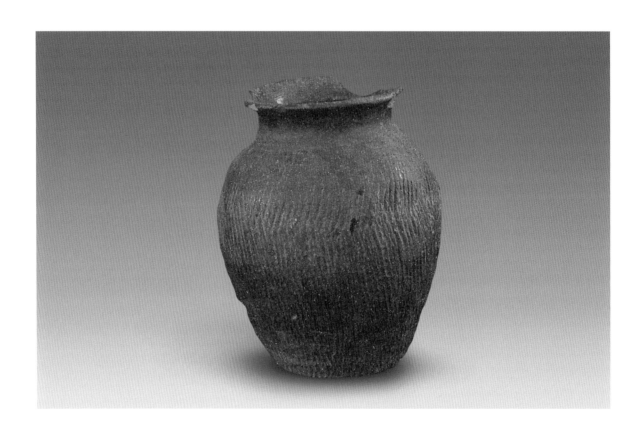

陶罐

汉

陶质

口径 11 厘米，底径 10 厘米，通高 8 厘米，重 1150 克

Pottery Jar

Han Dynasty

Pottery

Mouth Diameter 11 cm/ Bottom Diameter 10 cm/ Height 8 cm/ Weight 1,150 g

通体绳纹，口沿外卷，侈口直斜腹。口沿残两处。

盛贮器，生活用器具。陕西省鄠邑区征集。

陕西医史博物馆藏

This pottery jar is covered with cord pattern. It has a flared mouth with an everted rim and a slightly tapering body. There are two damaged areas on the mouth rim. The jar is a typical household storage utensil, and was collected from Huyi District, Shaanxi Province.

Preserved in Shaanxi Museum of Medical History

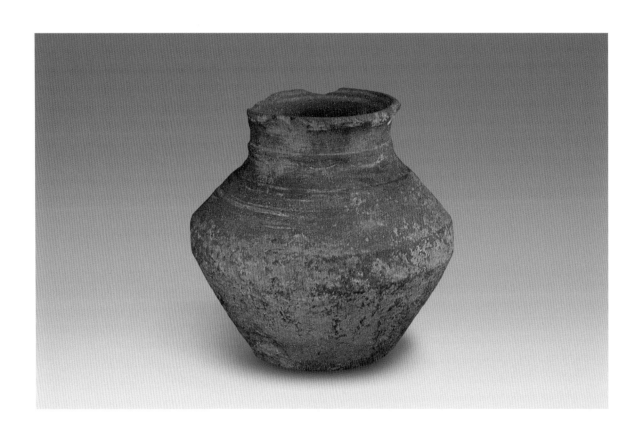

陶罐

汉

陶质

口径 8.5 厘米，底径 8 厘米，通高 13 厘米，重
800 克

灰陶，折肩，侈口，斜腹，平底。口沿残缺。盛
贮器，生活用器具。

陕西医史博物馆藏

Pottery Jar

Han Dynasty

Pottery

Mouth Diameter 8.5 cm/ Bottom Diameter 8 cm/
Height 13 cm/ Weight 800 g

This grey pottery jar has an angular shoulder, a
flared mouth, a tapering ovoid body and a flat
bottom. The mouth rim is damaged. It is a typical
household utensil for storage.

Preserved in Shaanxi Museum of Medical History

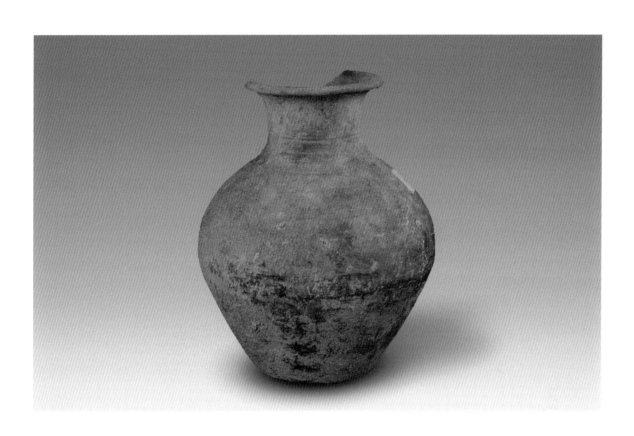

陶罐

汉

陶质

口径 10.5 厘米，底径 10 厘米，通高 21 厘米，

重 1500 克

圆腹，颈略高，喇叭口，平底。口沿残 3/5。盛贮器，

生活用器具。

陕西医史博物馆藏

Pottery Jar

Han Dynasty

Pottery

Mouth Diameter 10.5 cm/ Bottom Diameter 10 cm/

Height 21 cm/ Weight 1,500 g

This pottery jar has a rounded belly, a relatively

high neck, a trumpet-shaped mouth and a flat

bottom. Three fifths of the mouth rim is damaged. It

was used as a household utensil for storage.

Preserved in Shaanxi Museum of Medical History

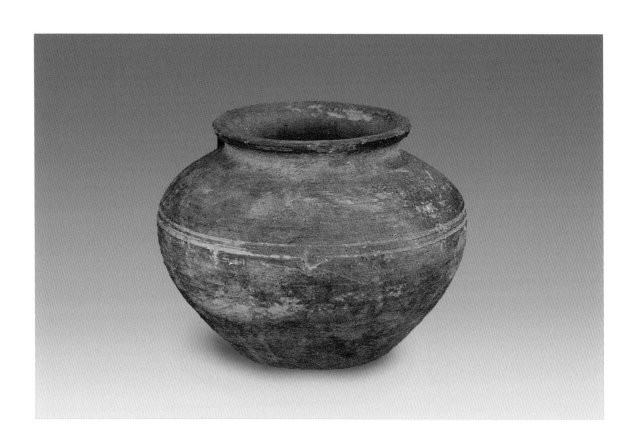

陶罐

汉

陶质

口径 12.5 厘米，底径 11 厘米，通高 13 厘米，
重 1250 克

扁腹，圆唇，平底。完整无损。盛贮器，生活用
器具。

陕西医史博物馆藏

Pottery Jar

Han Dynasty

Pottery

Mouth Diameter 12.5 cm/ Bottom Diameter 11 cm/
Height 13 cm/ Weight 1,250 g

This pottery jar has a compressed globular body, a
round rim and a flat bottom. The jar remains intact,
and was used as household storage utensil.

Preserved in Shaanxi Museum of Medical History

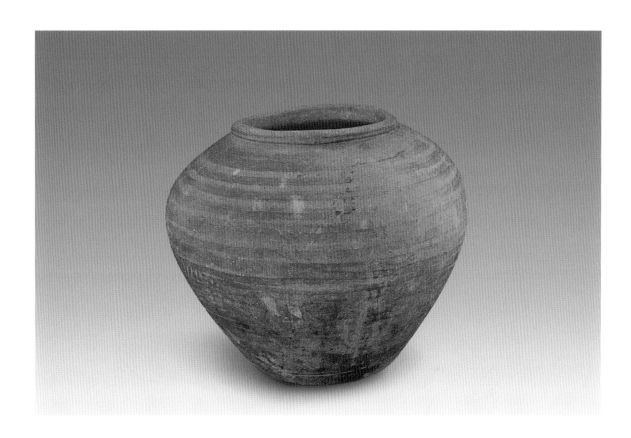

陶罐

汉

陶质

口径 15 厘米，底径 14 厘米，通高 20 厘米，重 3100 克

大口，条状纹，灰陶，圆唇，圆腹，平底。完整无损。盛贮器，生活用器具。

陕西医史博物馆藏

Pottery Jar

Han Dynasty

Pottery

Mouth Diameter 15 cm/ Bottom Diameter 14 cm/ Height 20 cm/ Weight 3,100 g

This grey pottery jar with stripe patterns features a wide mouth, a round rim, a rounded belly and a flat bottom. This jar remains intact and served as a household storage utensil.

Preserved in Shaanxi Museum of Medical History

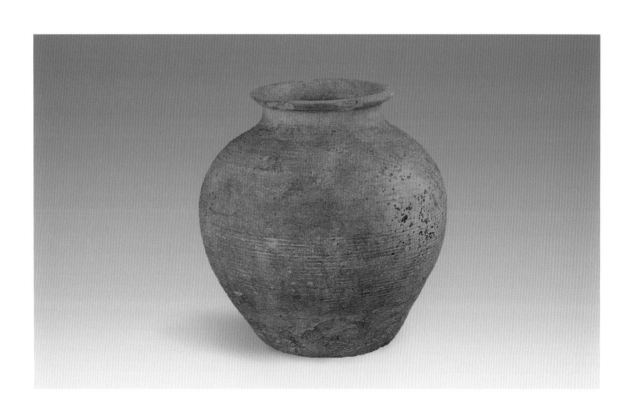

陶罐

汉

陶质

口径 11.5 厘米，底径 12.5 厘米，通高 19 厘米，
重 1800 克

圆唇，圆腹，细条纹，平底。口沿有残。盛贮器，
生活用器具。陕西省鄠邑区征集。

陕西医史博物馆藏

Pottery Jar

Han Dynasty

Pottery

Mouth Diameter 11.5 cm/ Bottom Diameter 12.5
cm/ Height 19 cm/ Weight 1,800 g

This pottery jar, the mouth rim of which is cracked,
features a circular rim, a rounded belly adorned
with thin stripe patterns, and a flat bottom. This
household utensil for storage was collected from
Huyi District, Shaanxi Province.

Preserved in Shaanxi Museum of Medical History

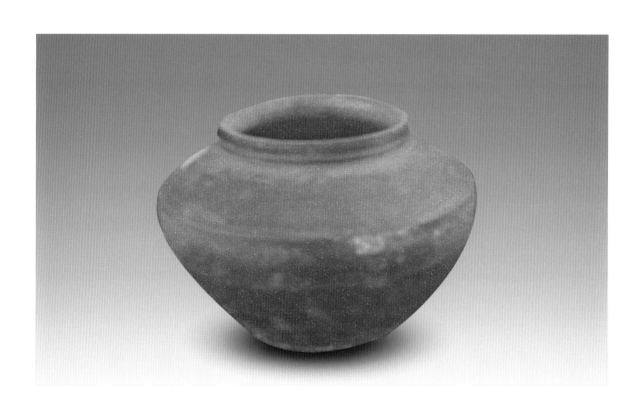

陶罐

汉

陶质

口径 12.5 厘米，底径 12 厘米，通高 13 厘米，
1050 克

黑色，折肩，直口，斜腹，平底。完整无损。盛
贮器，生活用器具。

陕西医史博物馆收藏

Pottery Jar

Han Dynasty

Pottery

Mouth Diameter 12.5 cm/ Bottom Diameter 12 cm/
Height 13 cm/ Weight 1,050 g

The black jar features a sloping shoulder, a straight
mouth, a tapering body, and a flat bottom. It remains
intact and served as a household storage utensil.

Preserved in Shaanxi Museum of Medical History

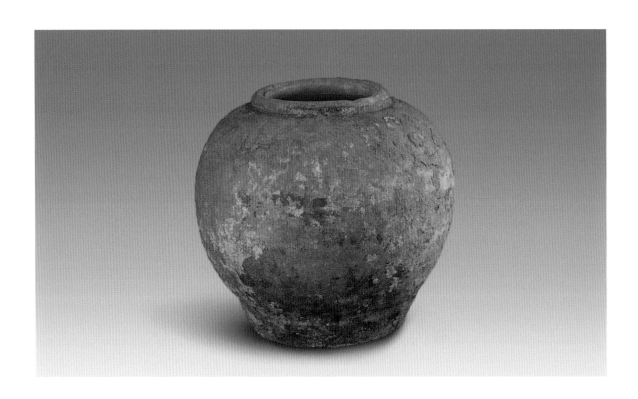

陶罐

汉

陶质

口径 9 厘米，底径 11 厘米，通高 15 厘米，重
1450 克

无颈，低口沿，圆口，圆腹，平底。盛贮器，生
活用器具。完整无损。陕西省鄠邑区征集。

陕西医史博物馆藏

Pottery Jar

Han Dynasty

Pottery

Mouth Diameter 9 cm/ Bottom Diameter 11 cm/
Height 15 cm/ Weight 1,450 g

This pottery jar has no neck but featuring a circular
mouth with a low mouth rim, a globular body,
and a flat bottom. It served as a household utensil
for storage. The jar has been kept intact and was
collected in Huyi District, Shaanxi Province.

Preserved in Shaanxi Museum of Medical History

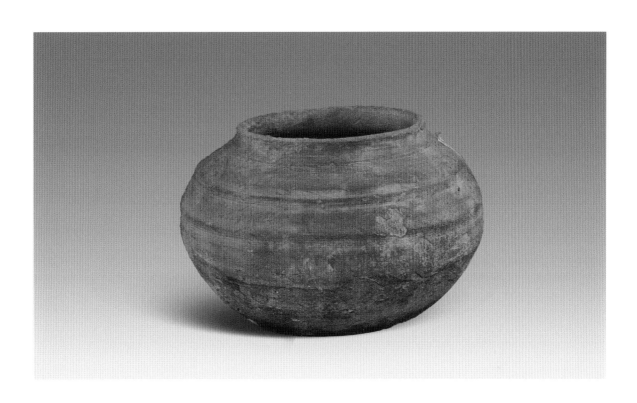

陶罐

汉

陶质

口径 12 厘米，底径 12 厘米，通高 12 厘米，重 1350 克

敞口，鼓腹，腹上有二道凸弦纹，平底。盛贮器，生活用器具。完整无损。陕西省澄城县善化乡征集。

陕西医史博物馆藏

Pottery Jar

Han Dynasty

Pottery

Mouth Diameter 12 cm/ Bottom Diameter 12 cm/ Height 12 cm/ Weight 1,350 g

This pottery jar has a everted mouth, a globular body with two bands of raised bowstring patterns and a flat bottom. The jar served as a household utensil for storage. It was collected from Shanhua Township in Chengcheng County, Shaanxi Province, and remains intact.

Preserved in Shaanxi Museum of Medical History

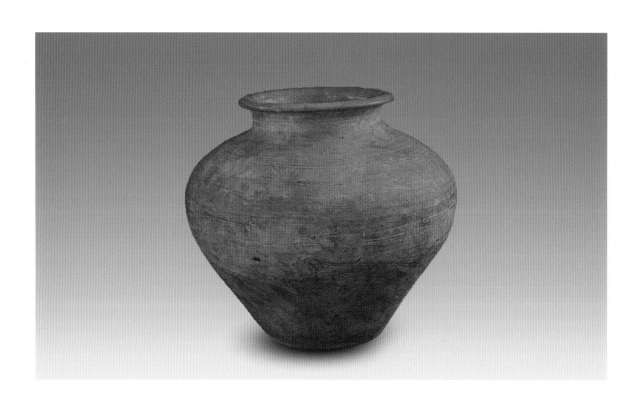

陶罐

汉

陶质

口径 14 厘米，底径 17 厘米，通高 21 厘米，重 2000 克

口沿外卷，喇叭口，折肩，平底。口沿有残。盛贮器，生活用器具。陕西省渭南市征集。

陕西医史博物馆藏

Pottery Jar

Han Dynasty

Pottery

Mouth Diameter 14 cm/ Bottom Diameter 17 cm/ Height 21 cm/ Weight 2,000 g

This pottery jar features a trumpet-shaped mouth with an everted rim, an angular shoulder and a flat bottom. The mouth rim is cracked. The jar served as a household utensil for storage, and was collected from Weinan City, Shaanxi Province.

Preserved in Shaanxi Museum of Medical History

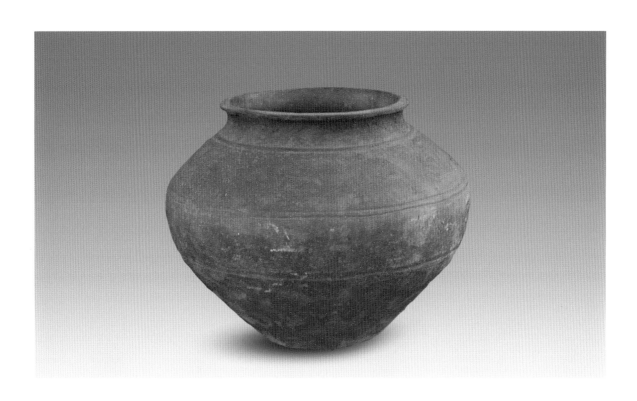

陶罐

汉

陶质

口径 16.5 厘米，底径 12 厘米，通高 20 厘米，
重 2200 克

敞口，腹部有环状纹，折肩，平底。口沿有残。
盛贮器，生活用器具。陕西省澄城县征集。

陕西医史博物馆藏

Pottery Jar

Han Dynasty

Pottery

Mouth Diameter 16.5 cm/ Bottom Diameter 12 cm/
Height 21 cm/ Weight 2,200 g

This pottery jar has a flared mouth, a belly which is
adorned with ring patterns, an angular shoulder and a
flat bottom.The mouth rim is cracked. The jar served
as a household utensil for storage, and was collected
from Chengcheng County, Shaanxi Province.

Preserved in Shaanxi Museum of Medical History

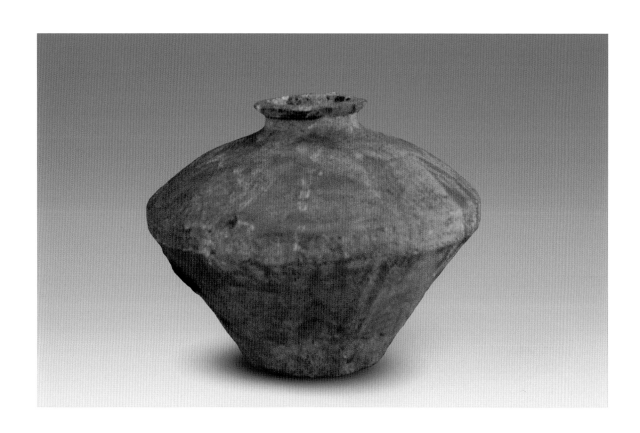

陶罐

汉

陶质

口径 12 厘米，底径 15.5 厘米，通高 22.5 厘米，
重 4400 克

平口沿，斜腹，折肩，平底。口沿有残。盛贮器，
生活用器具。

陕西医史博物馆藏

Pottery Jar

Han Dynasty

Pottery

Mouth Diameter 12 cm/ Bottom Diameter 15.5 cm/
Height 22.5 cm/ Weight 4,400 g

This pottery jar has a flat mouth rim, a tapering
ovoid body, an angular shoulder and a flat bottom.
The mouth rim is cracked. It was utilized as a
household utensil for storage.

Preserved in Shaanxi Museum of Medical History

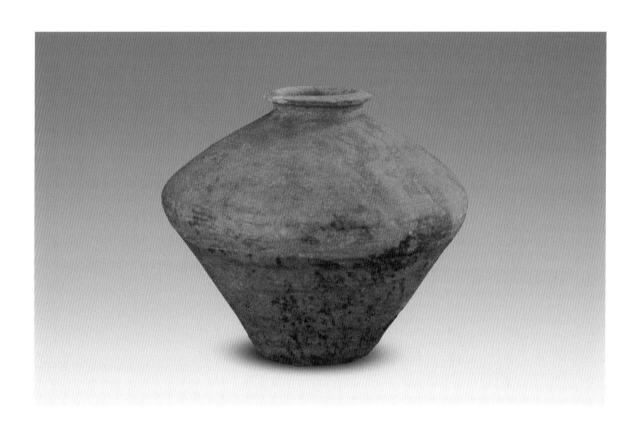

陶罐

汉

陶质

口径 13 厘米，底径 14 厘米，通高 28.5 厘米，
重 5000 克

喇叭口，折肩，斜腹，平底。肩部有一条状孔。

盛贮器，生活用器具。

陕西医史博物馆藏

Pottery Jar

Han Dynasty

Pottery

Mouth Diameter 13 cm/ Bottom Diameter 14 cm/
Height 28.5 cm/ Weight 5,000 g

This pottery jar has a trumpet-shaped mouth, an
angular shoulder, a tapering body and a flat bottom.
A bar-shaped hole can be seen on the shoulder. It
was used as a household utensil for storage.

Preserved in Shaanxi Museum of Medical History

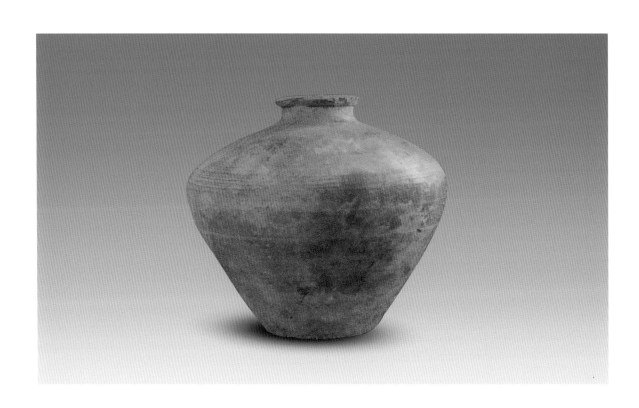

陶罐

汉

陶质

口径 12 厘米，底径 16 厘米，通高 30 厘米，重 4650 克

小口，折肩，有指甲纹，平口沿，平底。口沿有残。盛贮器，生活用器具。

陕西医史博物馆藏

Pottery Jar

Han Dynasty

Pottery

Mouth Diameter 12 cm/ Bottom Diameter 16 cm/ Height 30 cm/ Weight 4,650 g

This pottery jar has a narrow mouth, an angular shoulder decorated with patterns of fingernails, a flat mouth rim and a flat bottom. The mouth rim is cracked. It was utilized as a household utensil for storage.

Preserved in Shaanxi Museum of Medical History

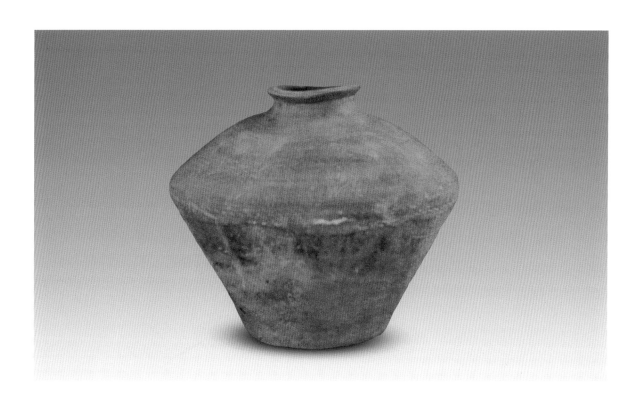

陶罐

汉

陶质

口径 10.5 厘米，底径 16.5 厘米，通高 26 厘米，
重 3900 克

小口，口沿不规则，折肩，有指纹，斜腹。口沿
有残。盛贮器，生活用器具。

陕西医史博物馆藏

Pottery Jar

Han Dynasty

Pottery

Mouth Diameter 10.5 cm/ Bottom Diameter 16.5
cm/ Height 26 cm/ Weight 3,900 g

This pottery jar has a narrow mouth, a rough mouth
rim, an angular shoulder with patterns of fingernails,
and a tapering body. The mouth rim is cracked. It
served as a household utensil for storage.

Preserved in Shaanxi Museum of Medical History

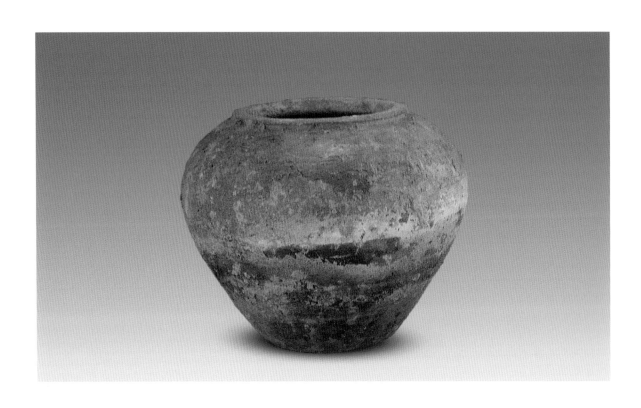

陶罐

汉

陶质

口径 15.5 厘米，底径 12.5 厘米，通高 18.5 厘米，
重 2500 克

无颈，无口沿，圆腹，平底。完整无损。盛贮器，
生活用器具。陕西省鄠邑区征集。

陕西医史博物馆藏

Pottery Jar

Han Dynasty

Pottery

Mouth Diameter 15.5 cm/ Bottom Diameter 12.5
cm/ Height 18.5 cm/ Weight 2,500 g

Without the neck and the mouth rim, this pottery
jar has a rounded belly and a flat bottom. It was
utilized as a household utensil for storage, and
remains intact. The jar was collected from Huyi
District, Shaanxi Province.

Preserved in Shaanxi Museum of Medical History

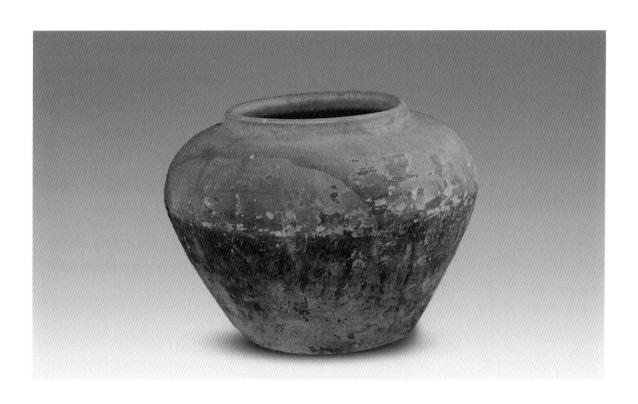

陶罐

汉

陶质

口径 18.5 厘米，底径 19 厘米，通高 21 厘米，
重 3350 克。

大口，折肩，无颈。完整无损。盛贮器，生活用
器具。陕西省鄠邑区征集。

陕西医史博物馆藏

Pottery Jar

Han Dynasty

Pottery

Mouth Diameter 18.5 cm/ Bottom Diameter 19 cm/
Height 21 cm/ Weight 3,350 g

This pottery jar has a wide mouth, an angular
shoulder with no neck. It was used as a household
utensil for storage. The well-preserved jar was
collected from Huyi District, Shaanxi Province.

Preserved in Shaanxi Museum of Medical History

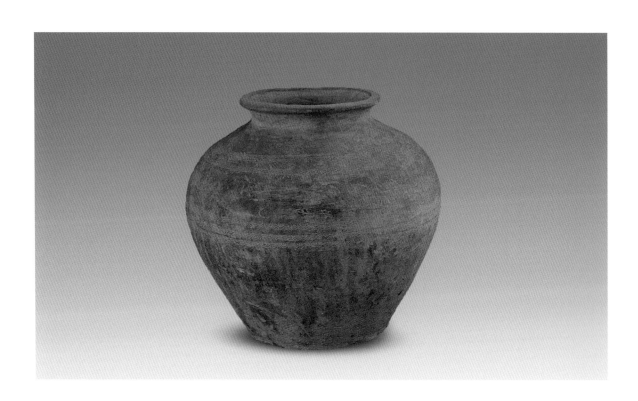

陶罐

汉

陶质

口径 15 厘米，底径 15.5 厘米，通高 23 厘米，重 2400 克

口沿外卷，细棱纹直口，圆腹，平底。完整无损。盛贮器，生活用器具。陕西省澄城县征集。

陕西医史博物馆藏

Pottery Jar

Han Dynasty

Pottery

Mouth Diameter 15 cm/ Bottom Diameter 15.5 cm/ Height 23 cm/ Weight 2,400 g

This pottery jar, which is adorned with delicate ribbed patterns, has an everted rim, a straight mouth, a globular body and a flat bottom. It was utilized as a household utensil for storage. The well-preserved jar was collected from Chengcheng County, Shaanxi Province.

Preserved in Shaanxi Museum of Medical History

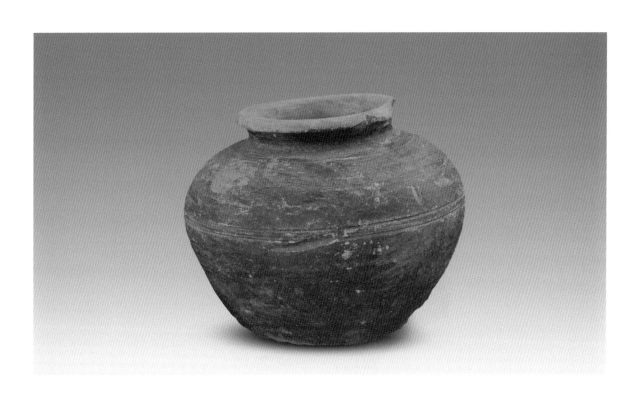

陶罐

汉

陶质

口径 10 厘米，底径 8.5 厘米，通高 13.0 厘米，
重 800 克

黑色，肩部有条纹，圆唇，圆腹，平底。口沿有
残。盛贮器，生活用器具。陕西省澄城县征集。

陕西医史博物馆藏

Pottery Jar

Han Dynasty

Pottery

Mouth Diameter 10 cm/ Bottom Diameter 8.5 cm/
Height 13.0 cm/ Weight 800 g

With stripe patterns on the shoulder, this black pottery
jar has a circular rim, a rounded belly and a flat
bottom. The mouth rim is cracked. The jar served as a
household utensil for storage, and was collected from
Chengcheng County, Shaanxi Province.

Preserved in Shaanxi Museum of Medical History

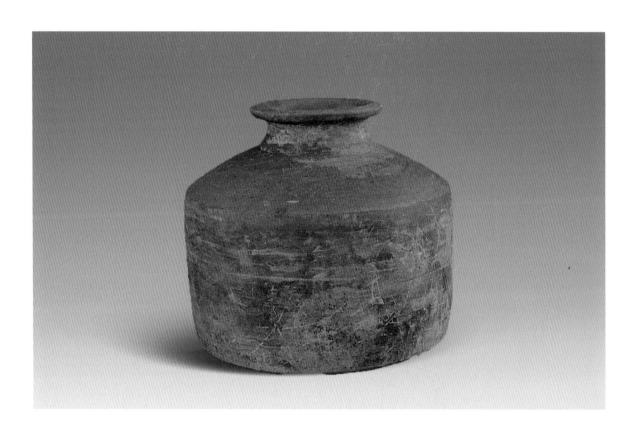

陶罐

汉

陶质

口径 12.5 厘米，底径 23.5 厘米，通高 20 厘米，重 3050 克

侈口，折肩，直腹，平底。完整无损。盛贮器，生活用器具。

陕西医史博物馆藏

Pottery Jar

Han Dynasty

Pottery

Mouth Diameter 12.5 cm/ Bottom Diameter 23.5 cm/ Height 20 cm/ Weight 3,050 g

This pottery jar features a flared mouth, an angular shoulder, a straight belly and a flat bottom. It was utilized as a household utensil for storage, and remains intact.

Preserved in Shaanxi Museum of Medical History

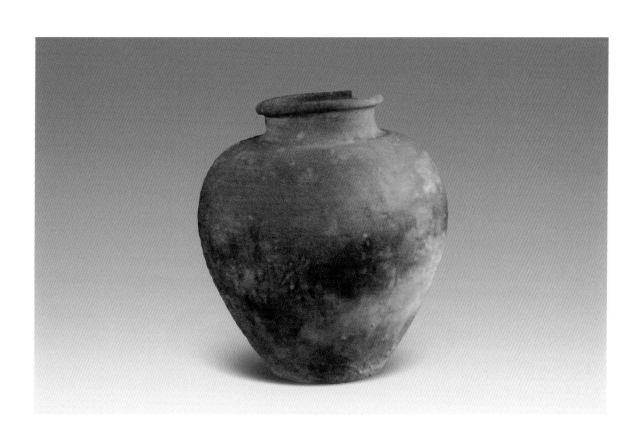

陶罐

汉

陶质

口径 13 厘米，底径 12 厘米，通高 26 厘米，重 2600 克

圆唇，圆腹，圆肩，平底。口沿有残。盛贮器，生活用器具。

陕西医史博物馆藏

Pottery Jar

Han Dynasty

Pottery

Mouth Diameter 13 cm/ Bottom Diameter 12 cm/ Height 26 cm/ Weight 2,600 g

This pottery jar has a circular rim, a globular body, a rounded shoulder and a flat bottom. The mouth rim is cracked. It was used as a household utensil for storage.

Preserved in Shaanxi Museum of Medical History

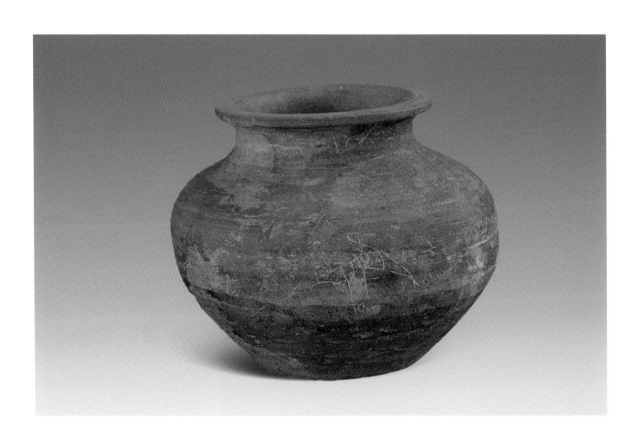

陶罐

汉

陶质

口径 9 厘米，底径 8 厘米，通高 11 厘米，重
600 克

口沿外卷，平口沿，鼓腹，平底。完整无损。盛
贮器，生活用器具。

陕西医史博物馆藏

Pottery Jar

Han Dynasty

Pottery

Mouth Diameter 9 cm/ Bottom Diameter 8 cm/
Height 11 cm/ Weight 600 g

This pottery jar has a flat mouth with an everted
rim, a globular body and a flat bottom. It is a well-
preserved household utensil for storage.

Preserved in Shaanxi Museum of Medical History

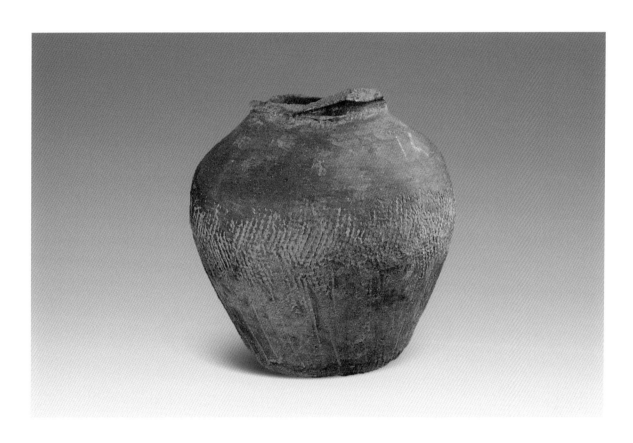

陶罐

汉

陶质

口径 11 厘米，底径 9.5 厘米，通高 16 厘米，
重 1000 克

腹部有锯齿纹。口沿全损。盛贮器，生活用器具。

陕西医史博物馆藏

Pottery Jar

Han Dynasty

Pottery

Mouth Diameter 11 cm/ Bottom Diameter 9.5 cm/
Height 16 cm/ Weight 1,000 g

This pottery jar is adorned with seesaw design
around the abdomen.The mouth rim is completely
damaged. It served as a household utensil for
storage.

Preserved in Shaanxi Museum of Medical History

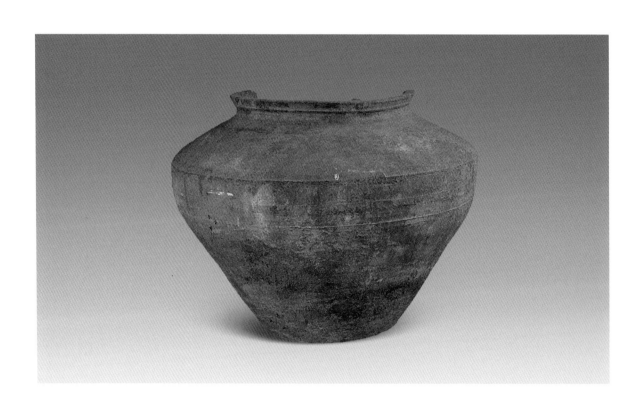

陶罐

汉

陶质

口径 20.5 厘米，底径 16 厘米，通高 23 厘米，
重 3700 克

侈口，折肩，斜腹，平底。口沿有残。盛贮器，
生活用器具。

陕西医史博物馆藏

Pottery Jar

Han Dynasty

Pottery

Mouth Diameter 20.5 cm/ Bottom Diameter 16 cm/
Height 23 cm/ Weight 3,700 g

This pottery jar has a wide flared mouth, an angular
shoulder, a tapering ovoid body and a flat bottom.
It served as a household utensil for storage, and its
mouth rim is cracked.

Preserved in Shaanxi Museum of Medical History

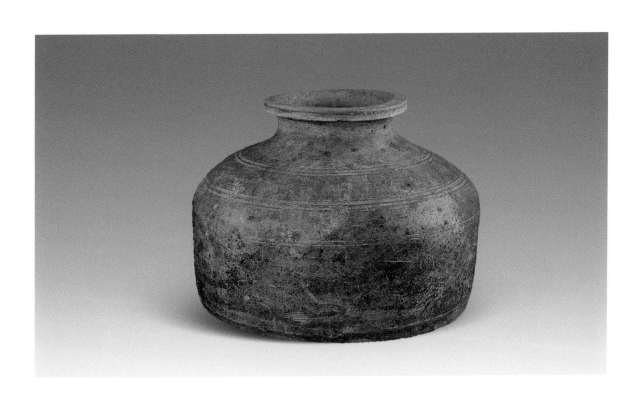

陶罐

汉

陶质

口径 11.5 厘米，底径 21.5 厘米，通高 14.5 厘米，重 2100 克

平口沿，直扁腹，平底。肩部有两道弦纹。口沿有残。盛贮器，生活用器具。

陕西医史博物馆藏

Pottery Jar

Han Dynasty

Pottery

Mouth Diameter 11.5 cm/ Bottom Diameter 21.5 cm/ Height 14.5 cm/ Weight 2,100 g

This pottery jar has a flat mouth rim, a domed body and a flat bottom. The shoulder is adorned with two bands of horizontal ring. The mouth rim is cracked. It served as a storage container for daily use.

Preserved in Shaanxi Museum of Medical History

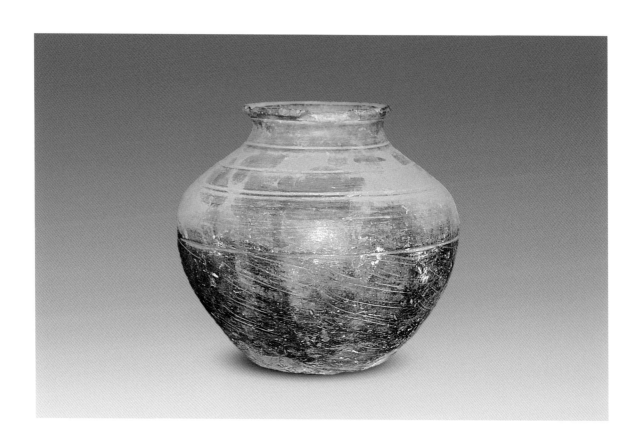

陶罐

汉

陶质

口径 10.3 厘米，底径 10.5 厘米，高 17.1 厘米，重 1400 克

Pottery Jar

Han Dynasty

Pottery

Mouth Diameter 10.3 cm/ Bottom Diameter 10.5 cm/ Height 17.1 cm/ Weight 1,400 g

子母口，溜肩，圆腹，平底，肩腹部有四道弦纹，
灰陶。口沿残。盛贮器。陕西省澄城县征集。

陕西医史博物馆藏

This grey pottery jar is designed with a buckle
lip, a sloping shoulder, a rounded abdomen,
and a flat bottom. There are four bands of
horizontal rings around the shoulder and
abdomen. The mouth rim is cracked. The jar
served as a storage container. and was collected
in Chengcheng County, Shaanxi Province.

Preserved in Shaanxi Museum of Medical History

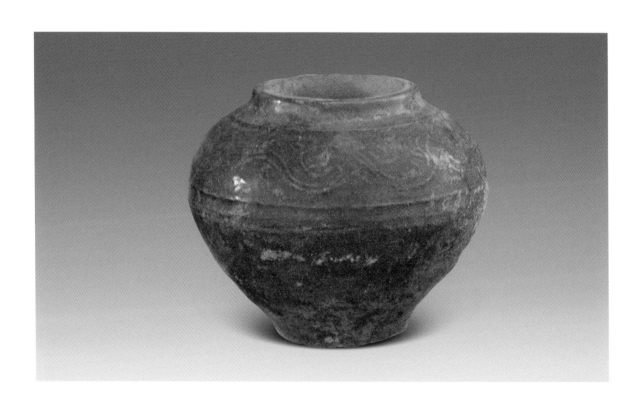

绿釉陶罐

汉

陶质

口径 8 厘米，底径 12.8 厘米，通高 7 厘米，重 1000 克

小圆口，圆肩，斜腹，平底，饰波浪纹。完整无损。盛贮器，生活用器具。

陕西医史博物馆藏

Green-glazed Pottery Jar

Han Dynasty

Pottery

Mouth Diameter 8 cm/ Bottom Diameter 12.8 cm/ Height 7 cm/ Weight 1,000 g

This jar has a small circular mouth, a rounded shoulder, a tapering ovoid body and a flat bottom. The jar is decorated with waviness ripple designs. It served as a storage container for daily use, and has been kept intact.

Preserved in Shaanxi Museum of Medical History

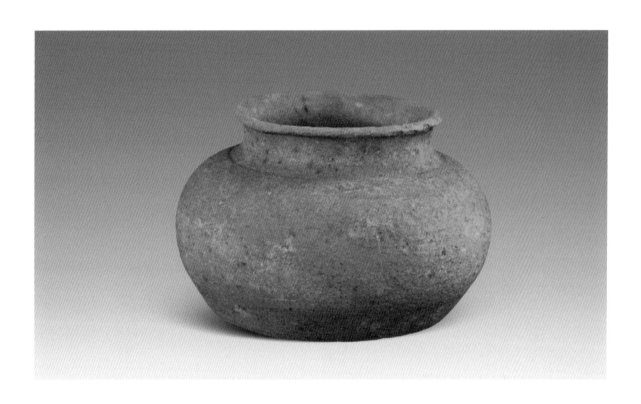

陶罐

汉

陶质

口径 10.5 厘米，底径 13 厘米，高 9.5 厘米，重 550 克

侈口，圆腹，平底。完整无损。盛贮器，生活用器具。

陕西医史博物馆藏

Pottery Jar

Han Dynasty

Pottery

Mouth Diameter 10.5 cm/ Bottom Diameter 13 cm/ Height 9.5 cm/ Weight 550 g

This pottery jar has a wide flared mouth, a rounded abdomen and a flat bottom. It served as a storage container for daily use, and has been kept in good condition.

Preserved in Shaanxi Museum of Medical History

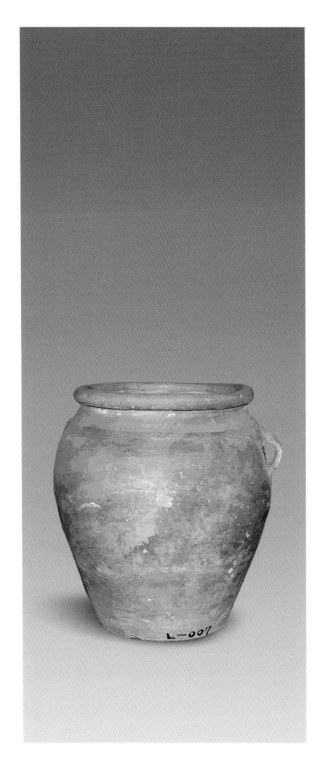

双耳陶罐

汉

陶质

口径 15 厘米，底径 11.4 厘米，高 19.7 厘米，
重 1450 克

Two-eared Pottery Jar

Han Dynasty

Pottery

Mouth Diameter 15 cm/ Bottom Diameter 11.4 cm/

Height 19.7 cm/ Weight 1,450 g

圆唇，圆肩，斜腹，平底，肩部有两耳，灰陶，素面。一耳残。生活器具。陕西省澄城县征集。

陕西医史博物馆藏

This pottery jar is designed with a circular mouth rim, a rounded shoulder with two ears attached, a tapering body and a flat bottom. One of the ears is damaged. This unglazed grey pottery jar was used as a household utensil for daily use, and was collected in Chengcheng County, Shaanxi Province.

Preserved in Shaanxi Museum of Medical History

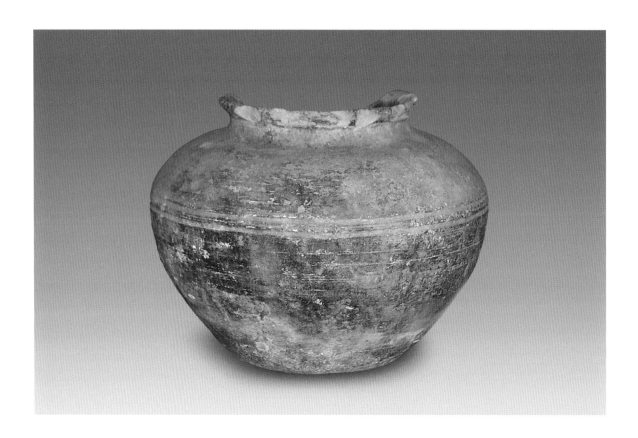

陶罐

汉

陶质

口径 12 厘米，底径 11 厘米，高 14.5 厘米，重 1250 克

Pottery Jar

Han Dynasty

Pottery

Mouth Diameter 12 cm/ Bottom Diameter 11 cm/ Height 14.5 cm/ Weight 1,250 g

侈口，圆肩，圆腹，平底，腹部有三道弦纹。
口残。盛贮器。陕西省澄城县征集。

陕西医史博物馆藏

This pottery jar has a wide flared mouth, a rounded shoulder, a globular body and a flat bottom. The abdomen is adorned with three bands of horizontal rings. The mouth is damaged. The jar served as a storage container, and was collected in Chengcheng County, Shaanxi Province.

Preserved in Shaanxi Museum of Medical History

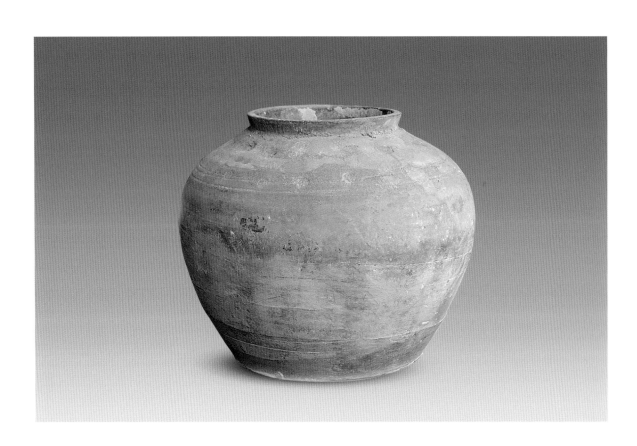

陶罐

汉

陶质

口径 12 厘米，底径 15.3 厘米，高 19.2 厘米，重 1500 克

Pottery Jar

Han Dynasty

Pottery

Mouth Diameter 12 cm/ Bottom Diameter 15.3 cm/ Height 19.2 cm/ Weight 1,500 g

直口，溜肩，圆腹，平底，灰陶，肩部有三道弦纹，
并有许多瓜果、蔬菜图案。完整无损。盛贮器。
陕西省澄城县团结村征集。

陕西医史博物馆藏

This grey pottery jar is designed with an upright
mouth, a sloping shoulder, a globular body and a
flat bottom. There are three bands of horizontal
rings and a variety of fruits and vegetable motifs
around the shoulder. It served as a storage
container and has been kept intact. The jar was
collected from Tuanjie Village of Chengcheng
County, Shaanxi Province.

Preserved in Shaanxi Museum of Medical History

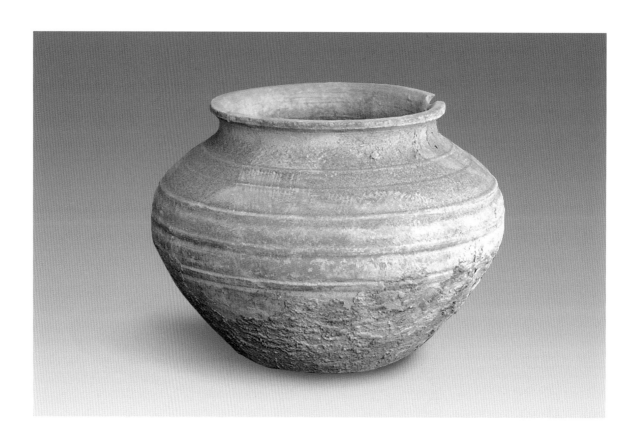

陶罐

汉

陶质

口径 12.5 厘米，底径 9.8 厘米，高 13 厘米

Pottery Jar

Han Dynasty

Pottery

Mouth Diameter 12.5 cm/ Bottom Diameter 9.8 cm/ Height 13 cm

圆唇，侈口，溜肩，圆腹，平底，肩腹部有
数道弦纹。口沿略残。盛贮器。陕西省澄城
县征集。

陕西医史博物馆藏

This pottery jar has a wide flared mouth with
a circular rim, a sloping shoulder, a rounded
abdomen and a flat bottom. The shoulder and
abdomen are decorated with a few rings of
horizontal Lines. The mouth rim is slightly
cracked. The jar served as a storage container,
and was collected in Chengcheng County,
Shaanxi Province.

Preserved in Shaanxi Museum of Medical History

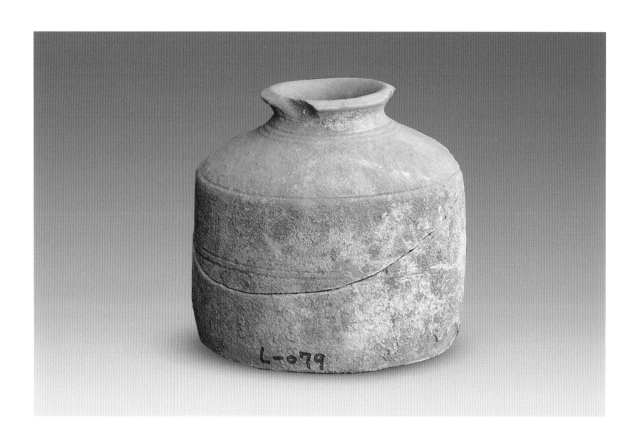

陶罐

汉

陶质

口径 7 厘米，底径 13.5 厘米，高 12.5 厘米，重 700 克

Pottery Jar

Han Dynasty

Pottery

Mouth Diameter 7 cm/ Bottom Diameter 13.5 cm/ Height 12.5 cm/ Weight 700 g

侈口，斜肩，直腹，平底，灰陶，腹部有二
道弦纹。有残。盛贮器。陕西省澄城县征集。

陕西医史博物馆藏

This grey pottery jar features a wide flared
mouth, a slant shoulder, a straight abdomen
and a flat bottom. There are two bands of
horizontal rings around the abdomen. The jar,
whose mouth is damaged, served as a storage
container. It was collected in Chengcheng
County, Shaanxi Province.
Preserved in Shaanxi Museum of Medical
History

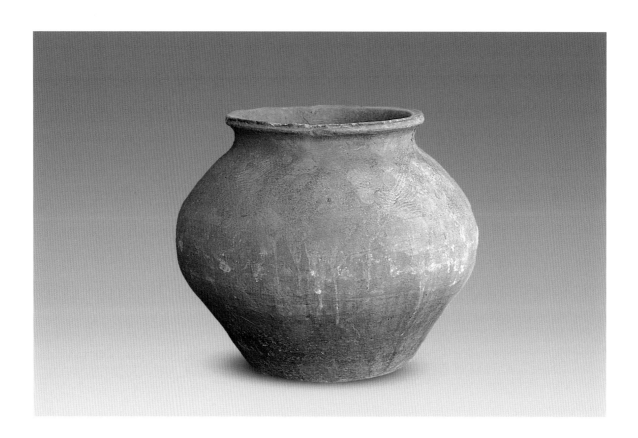

陶罐

汉

陶质

口径 17 厘米，底径 15.5 厘米，高 20.8 厘米，重 2500 克

Pottery Jar

Han Dynasty

Pottery

Mouth Diameter 17 cm/ Bottom Diameter 15.5 cm/ Height 20.8 cm/ Weight 2,500 g

侈口，溜肩，圆腹，平底，灰陶，底部有一圆孔。
口沿稍残。盛贮器。陕西省澄城县征集。

陕西医史博物馆藏

This grey pottery jar has a wide flared mouth, a sloping shoulder, a rounded belly and a flat bottom with a circular hole in it. It served as a storage container and the mouth rim is slightly cracked. It was collected in Chengcheng County, Shaanxi Province.

Preserved in Shaanxi Museum of Medical History

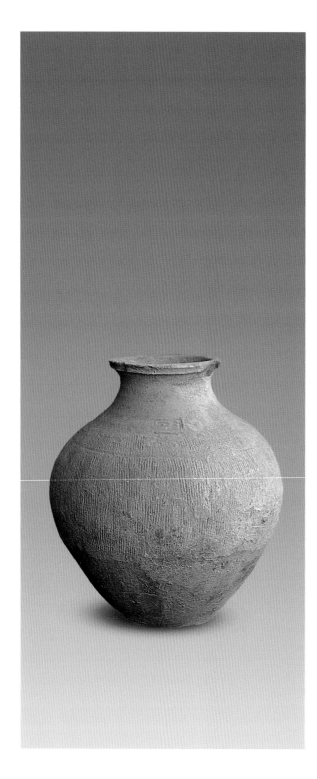

陶罐

汉

陶质

口径 10.5 厘米，底径 9.6 厘米，高 23 厘米，重 1900 克

Pottery Jar

Han Dynasty

Pottery

Mouth Diameter 10.5 cm/ Bottom Diameter 9.6 cm/

Height 23 cm/ Weight 1,900 g

平口沿，溜肩，圆腹，平底，肩部有一印记，
上腹为细绳纹。口沿残，下腹有裂纹。盛贮器。
陕西省澄城县征集。

陕西医史博物馆藏

This pottery jar has a flat mouth rim, a sloping
shoulder, a rounded belly and a flat bottom.
A marking can be found on the shoulder and
some thin cord patterns on the upper part of the
belly. There are cracks on the mouth rim and
the lower part of the belly. It served as a storage
container, and was collected in Chengcheng
County, Shaanxi Province.

Preserved in Shaanxi Museum of Medical History

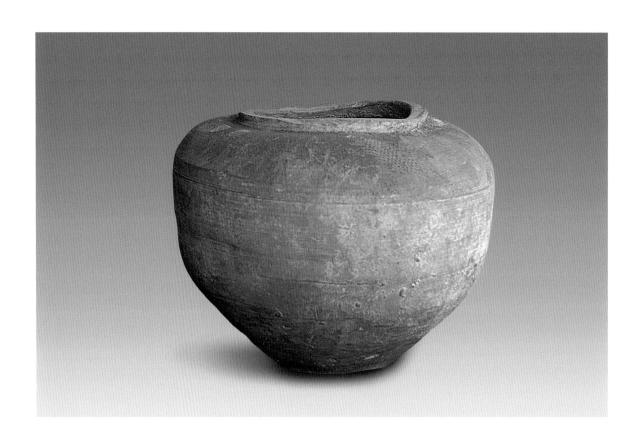

陶罐

汉

陶质

口径 13.5 厘米，底径 9.6 厘米，高 17.6 厘米，重 2150 克

Pottery Jar

Han Dynasty

Pottery

Mouth Diameter 13.5 cm/ Bottom Diameter 9.6 cm/ Height 17.6 cm/ Weight 2,150 g

圆口，平肩，直腹，平底，灰陶。完整无损。
盛贮器。陕西省澄城县征集。

陕西医史博物馆藏

This grey pottery jar is designed with a round
mouth, a flat shoulder, a straight abdomen
and a flat bottom. The jar served as a storage
container and has been kept in good condition.
It was collected in Chengcheng County, Shaanxi
Province.

Preserved in Shaanxi Museum of Medical
History

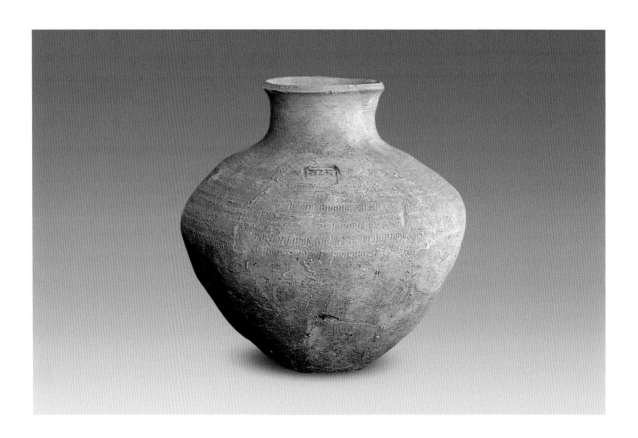

陶罐

汉

陶质

口径 9.8 厘米，底径 10.5 厘米，高 22 厘米，重 2050 克

Pottery Jar

Han Dynasty

Pottery

Mouth Diameter 9.8 cm/ Bottom Diameter 10.5 cm/ Height 22 cm/ Weight 2,050 g

侈口，短颈，溜肩，折腹，肩部有一印记，上腹部为短绳纹，灰陶。完整无损。盛贮器。陕西省澄城县征集。

陕西医史博物馆藏

This grey pottery jar has a wide flared mouth, a short neck, a sloping shoulder and a tapering ovoid body. A marking can be seen on the shoulder and some short sequences in chord patterns on the upper part of the belly. The jar served as a storage container and has been kept in good condition. It was collected in Chengcheng County, Shaanxi Province.
Preserved in Shaanxi Museum of Medical History

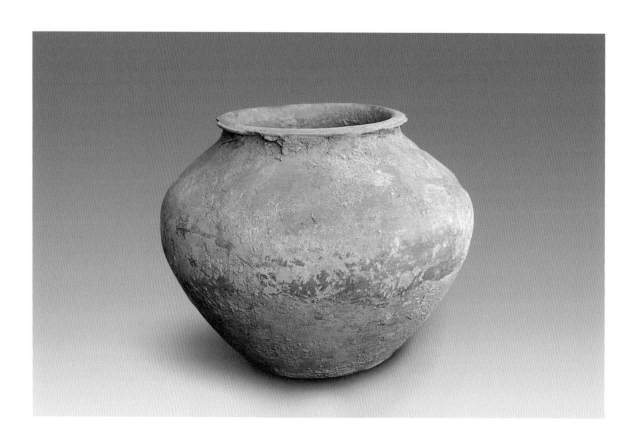

陶罐

汉

陶质

口径 15 厘米，底径 12 厘米，高 19.6 厘米，重 2250 克

Pottery Jar

Han Dynasty

Pottery

Mouth Diameter 15 cm/ Bottom Diameter 12 cm/ Height 19.6 cm/ Weight 2,250 g

圆唇，溜肩，圆腹，平底，灰陶，素面。完
整无损。盛贮器。陕西省澄城县征集。

陕西医史博物馆藏

This unglazed grey pottery jar is designed
with a round mouth rim, a sloping shoulder, a
globular body and a flat bottom. It served as a
storage container and remains intact. The jar
was collected in Chengcheng County, Shaanxi
Province.

Preserved in Shaanxi Museum of Medical History

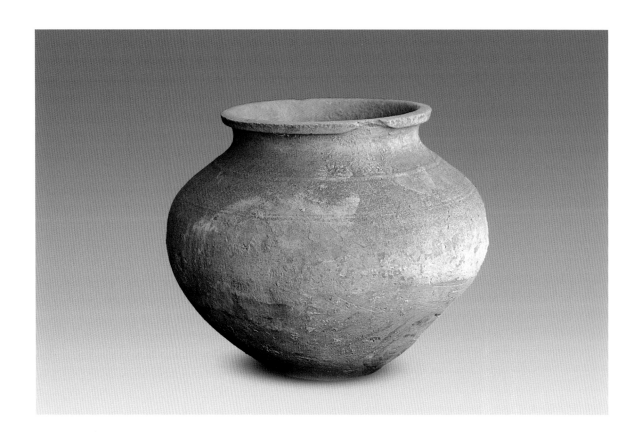

陶罐

汉

陶质

口径 16.6 厘米，底径 11.2 厘米，高 20 厘米，重 2150 克

Pottery Jar

Han Dynasty

Pottery

Mouth Diameter 16.6 cm/ Bottom Diameter 11.2 cm/ Height 20 cm/ Weight 2,150 g

圆唇，溜肩，圆腹，平底，肩部两道弦纹，灰陶。
口沿略残。盛贮器。陕西省澄城县征集。

陕西医史博物馆藏

This grey pottery jar is designed with a round
mouth rim, a sloping shoulder, a globular
body, and a flat bottom. There are two bands
of horizontal rings around the shoulder. The
jar served as a storage container and the mouth
rim is slightly cracked. It was collected in
Chengcheng County, Shaanxi Province.

Preserved in Shaanxi Museum of Medical History

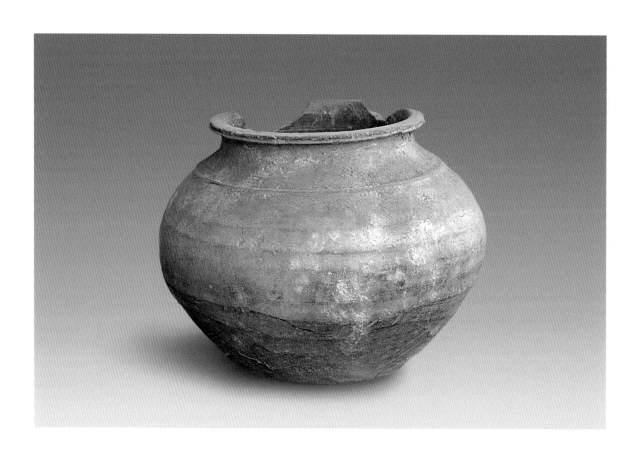

陶罐

汉

陶质

口径 14.5 厘米，底径 12.5 厘米，高 16 厘米，重 1400 克

Pottery Jar

Han Dynasty

Pottery

Mouth Diameter 14.5 cm/ Bottom Diameter 12.5 cm/ Height 16 cm/ Weight 1,400 g

圆唇，溜肩，圆腹，平底，肩部有一道凸棱，

灰陶。口沿残。盛贮器。陕西省澄城县征集。

陕西医史博物馆藏

This grey pottery jar features a round mouth rim, a sloping shoulder, a swelling belly, and a flat bottom. There is a raised band around the shoulder. The jar served as a storage container and the mouth rim is damaged. It was collected in Chengcheng County, Shaanxi Province.

Preserved in Shaanxi Museum of Medical History

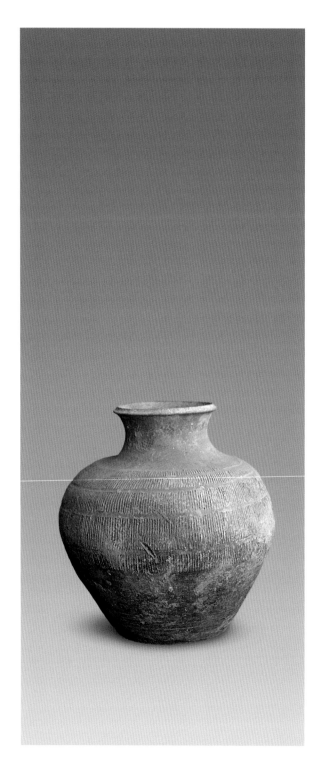

陶罐

汉

陶质

口径 11 厘米，底径 12 厘米，高 23.7 厘米，重 1800 克

Pottery Jar

Han Dynasty

Pottery

Mouth Diameter 11 cm/ Bottom Diameter 12 cm/ Height 23.7 cm/ Weight 1,800 g

侈口，平肩，圆腹，平底，上腹部为绳纹，灰陶。
完整无损。盛贮器。陕西省澄城县征集。

陕西医史博物馆藏

This grey pottery jar features a wide flared mouth, a flat shoulder, a rounded belly and a flat bottom. The upper part of the belly is adorned with cord patterns. The jar served as a storage container and remains intact. It was collected in Chengcheng County, Shaanxi Province.

Preserved in Shaanxi Museum of Medical History

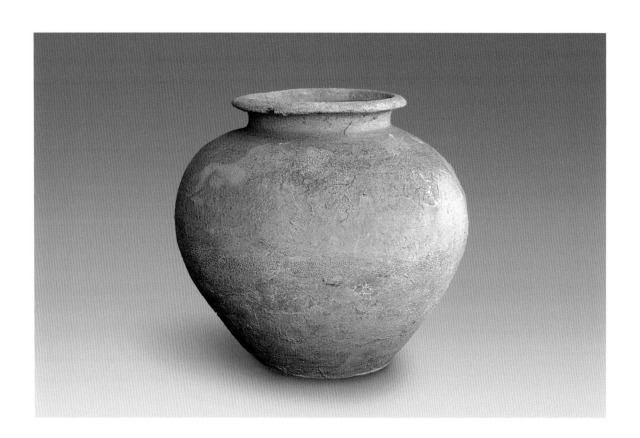

陶罐

汉

陶质

口径 14 厘米，底径 11.8 厘米，高 21 厘米，重 1700 克

Pottery Jar

Han Dynasty

Pottery

Mouth Diameter 14 cm/ Bottom Diameter 11.8 cm/ Height 21 cm/ Weight 1,700 g

圆唇，圆腹，平底，肩腹部有三道纹饰，灰陶。
完整无损。盛贮器。陕西省澄城县征集。

陕西医史博物馆藏

This grey pottery jar has a round mouth
rim, a swelling belly and a flat bottom. There
are three bands of horizontal rings around the
shoulder and belly. The jar served as a storage
container and remains intact. It was collected in
Chengcheng County, Shaanxi Province.

Preserved in Shaanxi Museum of Medical History

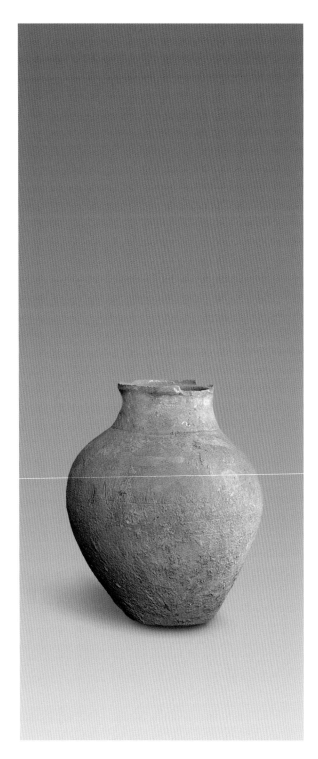

陶罐

汉

陶质

口径 10.6 厘米，底径 10 厘米，高 24.5 厘米，
重 2000 克

Pottery Jar

Han Dynasty

Pottery

Mouth Diameter 10.6 cm/ Bottom Diameter 10 cm/

Height 24.5 cm/ Weight 2,000 g

盘口，短颈，溜肩，圆腹，平底。腹上部为绳纹，

灰陶。口沿残。盛贮器。陕西省澄城县征集。

陕西医史博物馆藏

This grey pottery jar is designed with a dish-shaped mouth, a short neck, a sloping shoulder, a swelling belly, and a flat bottom. Cord patterns can be seen on the upper part of the belly. The mouth rim is damaged. The jar served as a storage container, and was collected in Chengcheng County, Shaanxi Province.

Preserved in Shaanxi Museum of Medical History

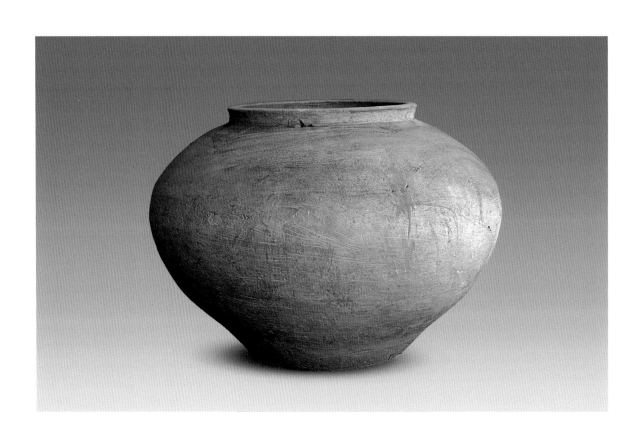

陶罐

汉

陶质

口径 24.3 厘米，底径 21 厘米，高 32 厘米，重
8400 克

平口沿，溜肩，圆腹，平底，灰陶，素面。完整
无损。盛贮器。

陕西医史博物馆藏

Pottery Jar

Han Dynasty

Pottery

Mouth Diameter 24.3 cm/ Bottom Diameter 21 cm/
Height 32 cm/ Weight 8,400 g

This unglazed grey pottery jar has a flat mouth
rim, a sloping shoulder, a rounded belly and a flat
bottom. The jar served as a storage container and
remains intact.

Preserved in Shaanxi Museum of Medical History

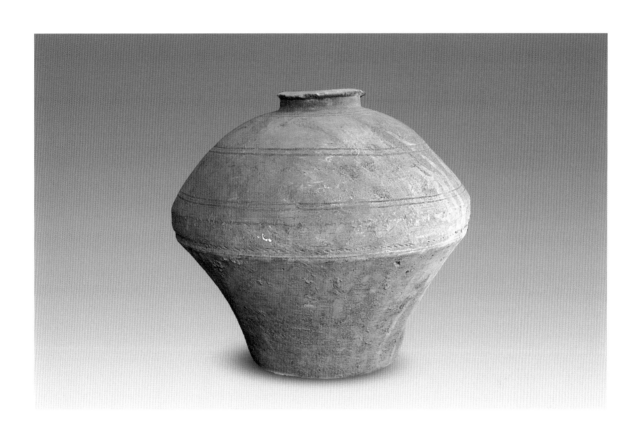

陶罐

汉

陶质

口径 14 厘米，底径 24 厘米，高 40 厘米，重 1040 克

平口沿，圆肩，折腹，平底，肩部有三道双弦纹。口沿残。盛贮器。

陕西医史博物馆藏

Pottery Jar

Han Dynasty

Pottery

Mouth Diameter 14 cm/ Bottom Diameter 24 cm/ Height 40 cm/ Weight 1,040 g

This pottery jar has a flat mouth rim, a rounded shoulder, a tapering ovoid body and a flat bottom. There are three sets of double horizontal rings around the shoulder. The mouth rim is cracked. The jar served as a storage container.

Preserved in Shaanxi Museum of Medical History

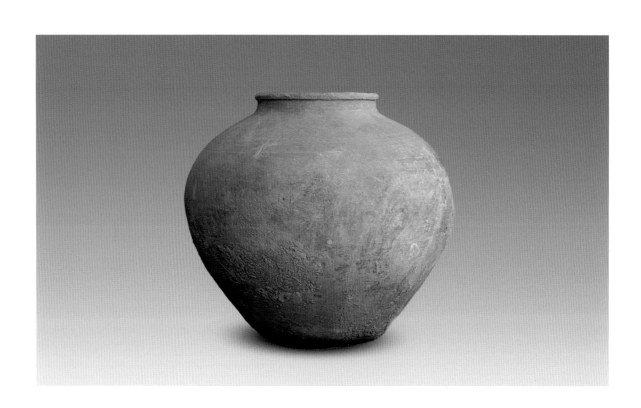

陶罐

汉

陶质

口径 18.5 厘米，底径 18 厘米，高 34.5 厘米。

重 5400 克

圆唇，溜肩，圆腹，平底，灰陶，肩部三道纹。

完整无损。盛贮器。

陕西医史博物馆藏

Pottery Jar

Han Dynasty

Pottery

Mouth Diameter 18.5 cm/ Bottom Diameter 18 cm/ Height 34.5 cm/ Weight 5,400 g

This grey pottery jar is designed with a circular mouth rim, a sloping shoulder, a swelling belly and a flat bottom. There are three bands of string patterns around the shoulder. The jar served as a storage container and remains intact.

Preserved in Shaanxi Museum of Medical History

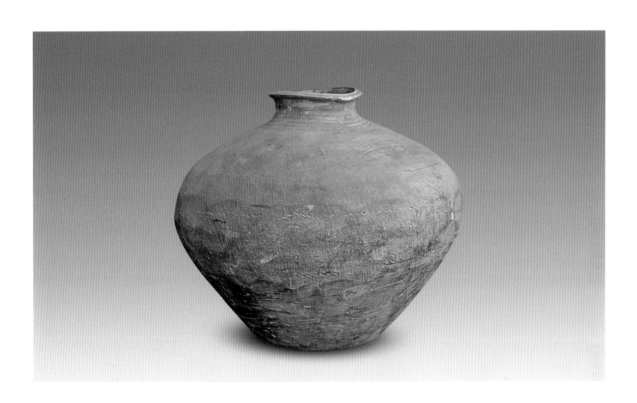

陶罐

汉

陶质

口径 11 厘米，底径 14.4 厘米，高 28 厘米，重 4300 克

圆唇，折腹，平底，肩部数道弦纹。完整无损。盛贮器。

陕西医史博物馆藏

Pottery Jar

Han Dynasty

Pottery

Mouth Diameter 11 cm/ Bottom Diameter 14.4 cm/ Height 28 cm/ Weight 4,300 g

This pottery jar features a circular mouth rim, a tapering ovoid body and a flat bottom. There are several bands of string patterns around the shoulder. The jar served as a storage container and remains intact.

Preserved in Shaanxi Museum of Medical History

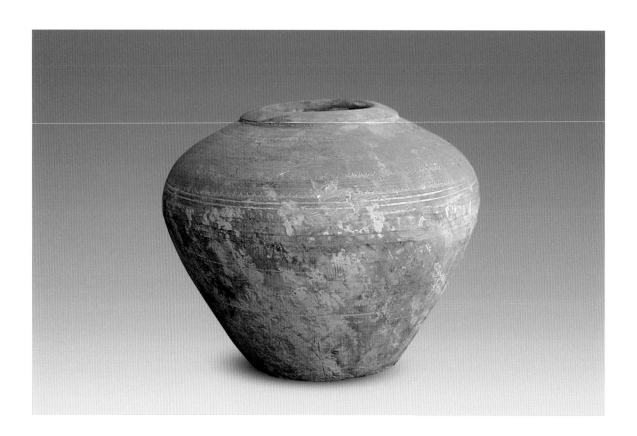

陶罐

汉

陶质

口径 10 厘米，底径 16.5 厘米，高 26.8 厘米。重 5900 克

Pottery Jar

Han Dynasty

Pottery

Mouth Diameter 10 cm/ Bottom Diameter 16.5 cm/ Height 26.8 cm/ Weight 5,900 g

平斜口沿，折腹，平底，肩部四圈波浪纹夹
杂有不同的圆形纹饰。腹部有一洞。盛贮器。
陕西省白水县征集。

陕西医史博物馆藏

This pottery jar has an inclined mouth rim, a
tapering ovoid body and a flat bottom. There
are four bands of waviness ripples mixed with
different types of circular patterns around the
shoulder. A hole can be found on the belly. The jar
served as a storage container, and was collected
from Baishui County, Shaanxi Province.
Preserved in Shaanxi Museum of Medical History

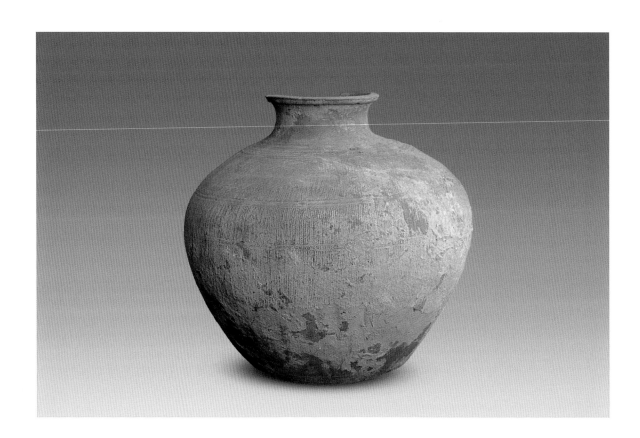

陶罐

汉

陶质

口径 11.2 厘米，底径 14.5 厘米，高 26.5 厘米，重 3350 克

Pottery Jar

Han Dynasty

Pottery

Mouth Diameter 11.2 cm/ Bottom Diameter 14.5 cm/ Height 26.5 cm/ Weight 3,350 g

圆唇，圆腹，平底，灰陶，肩部数道弦纹，并有一印记，腹为绳纹。口沿残。盛贮器。陕西省澄城县征集。

陕西医史博物馆藏

This grey pottery jar is designed with a circular mouth rim, a swelling belly and a flat bottom. There are a few bands of string patterns and a marking on the shoulder. The abdomen is adorned with cord patterns.The mouth rim is cracked. The jar served as a storage container, and was collected from Chengcheng County, Shaanxi Province.

Preserved in Shaanxi Museum of Medical History

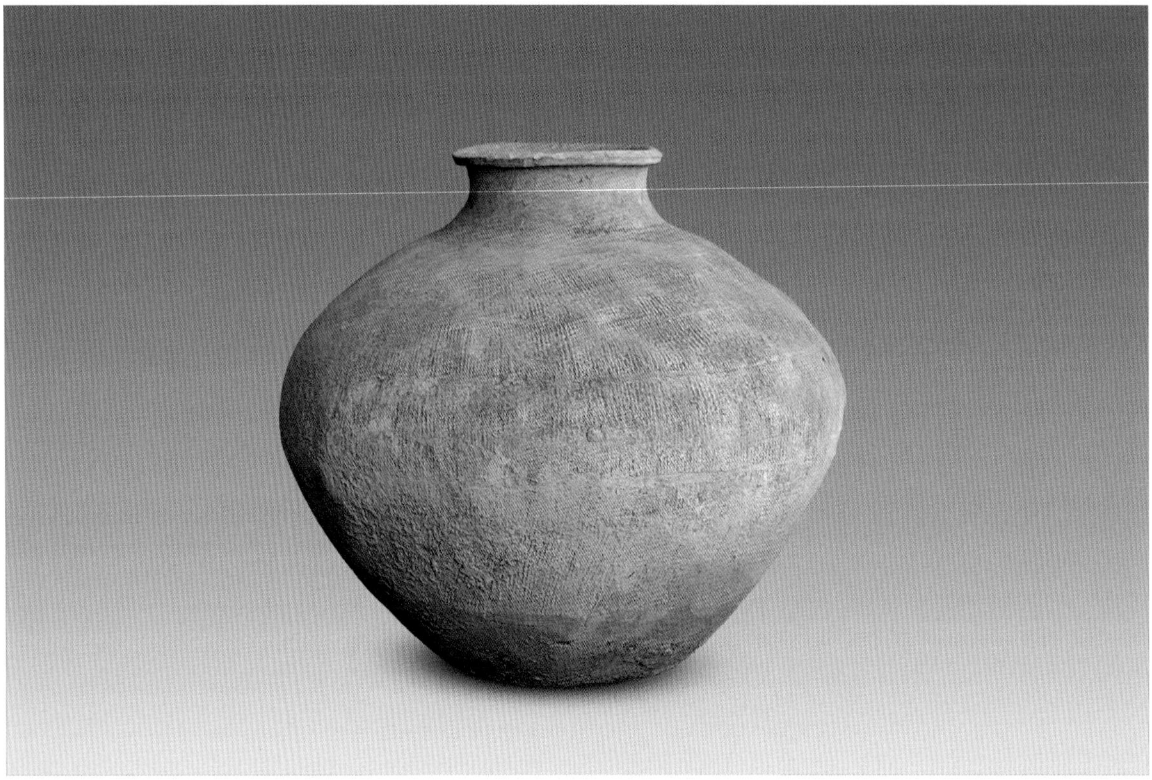

陶罐

汉

陶质

口径 11.3 厘米，底径 27 厘米，高 15 厘米，重 3000 克

Pottery Jar

Han Dynasty

Pottery

Mouth Diameter 11.3 cm/ Bottom Diameter 27 cm/ Height 15 cm/ Weight 3,000 g

圆唇，圆腹，平底，灰陶，肩部数道弦纹，腹为绳纹。完整无损。盛贮器。陕西省澄城县征集。

陕西医史博物馆藏

This grey pottery jar features a circular mouth rim, a swelling belly and a flat bottom. There are a few bands of string patterns around the shoulder and cord patterns around the belly. The jar served as a storage container and remains intact, and was collected from Chengcheng County, Shaanxi Province.

Preserved in Shaanxi Museum of Medical History

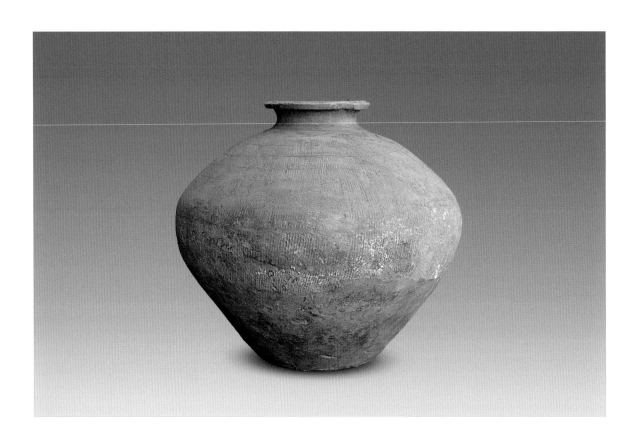

陶罐

汉

陶质

口径 11.8 厘米，底径 14 厘米，高 27.5 厘米，重 3300 克

Pottery Jar

Han Dynasty

Pottery

Mouth Diameter 11.8 cm/ Bottom Diameter 14 cm/ Height 27.5 cm/ Weight 3,300 g

圆唇，溜肩，折腹，平底，灰陶，细绳纹，夹有数道弦纹。完整无损。盛贮器。陕西省澄城县征集。

陕西医史博物馆藏

The grey pottery jar features a circular mouth rim, a sloping shoulder, a tapering ovoid body and a flat bottom. There are thin cord patterns mixed with a few bands of string patterns on the surface. The jar served as a storage container and remains intact. It was collected from Chengcheng County, Shaanxi Province.

Preserved in Shaanxi Museum of Medical History

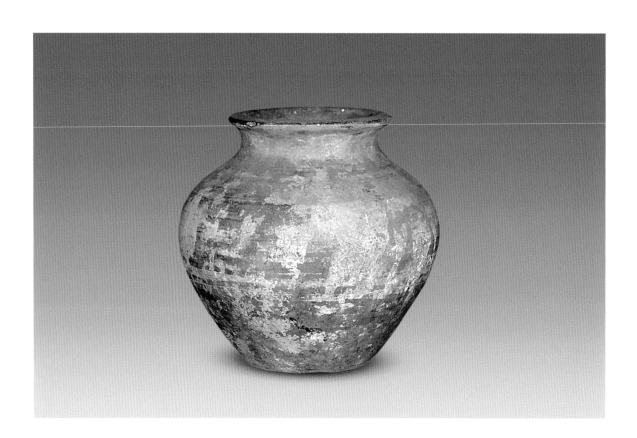

陶罐

汉

陶质

口径 10.5 厘米，底径 8.8 厘米，高 15.5 厘米，重 1100 克

Pottery Jar

Han Dynasty

Pottery

Mouth Diameter 10.5 cm/ Bottom Diameter 8.8 cm/ Height 15.5 cm/ Weight 1,100 g

平口沿，圆腹，平底，素面，灰陶。罐内有粟。
完整无损。盛贮器。陕西省澄城县征集。

陕西医史博物馆藏

This unglazed grey pottery jar has a flat mouth
rim, a rounded belly and a flat bottom. Some
willet grains can be found in the jar. The jar
served as a storage container, and remains
intact. It was collected from Chengcheng
County, Shaanxi Province.

Preserved in Shaanxi Museum of Medical History

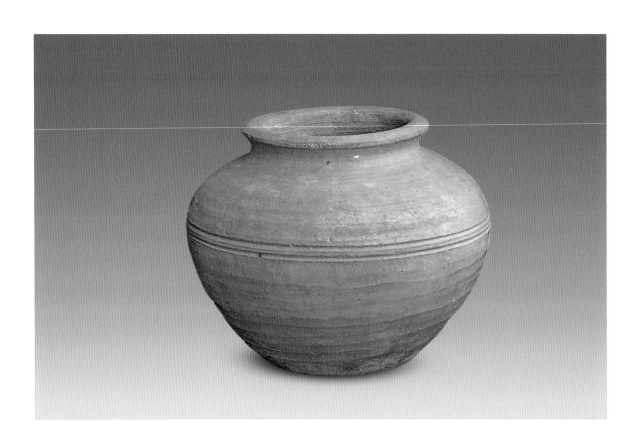

陶罐

汉

陶质

口径 10 厘米，底径 9 厘米，高 12.9 厘米，重 800 克

Pottery Jar

Han Dynasty

Pottery

Mouth Diameter 10 cm/ Bottom Diameter 9 cm/ Height 12.9 cm/ Weight 800 g

圆唇，圆腹，平底。上腹部有二道弦纹，灰陶，素面。完整无损。盛贮器。陕西省澄城县征集。

陕西医史博物馆藏

This unglazed grey pottery jar has a circular rim, a globular body and a flat bottom. There are a two bands of string patterns on the upper part of the belly. The jar served as a storage container and remains intact. It was collected from Chengcheng County, Shaanxi Province.

Preserved in Shaanxi Museum of Medical History

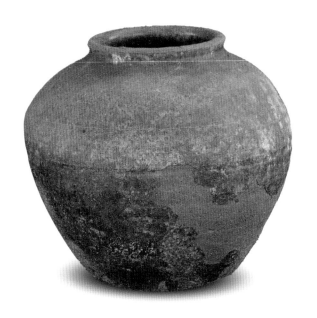

陶罐

汉

陶质

口径 8 厘米，底径 8.5 厘米，通高 13 厘米，重 1400 克

圆唇口，鼓腹，平底，黄釉色。完整无损。容器。陕西省西安市长安区康申利上交征集。

陕西医史博物馆藏

Pottery Jar

Han Dynasty

Pottery

Mouth Diameter 8 cm/ Bottom Diameter 8.5 cm/ Height 13 cm/ Weight 1,400 g

This yellow-glazed jar has a circular mouth rim, a globular body and a flat bottom. The jar served as a container and remains intact. It was donated by Kang Shenli from Chang'an District, Xi'an City, Shaanxi Province.

Preserved in Shaanxi Museum of Medical History

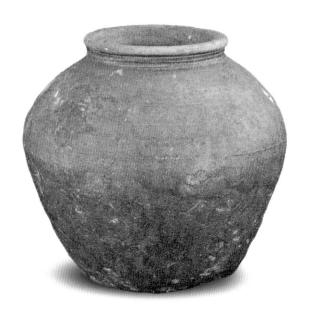

陶罐

汉

棕釉陶质

口径 8.5 厘米，底径 9 厘米，高 13 厘米，重 1510 克

圆唇口，鼓腹，平底，棕釉色。完整无损。明器，贮藏器具。陕西省西安市长安区康申利上交征集。

陕西医史博物馆藏

Pottery Jar

Han Dynasty

Brown-glazed Pottery

Mouth Diameter 8.5 cm/ Bottom Diameter 9 cm/ Height 13 cm/ Weight 1,510 g

This brown glazed pottery jar has a circular mouth rim, a globular body and a flat bottom. The jar is a burial object used for storage, and remains intact. It was donated by Kang Shenli from Chang'an District, Xi'an City Shaanxi Province.

Preserved in Shaanxi Museum of Medical History

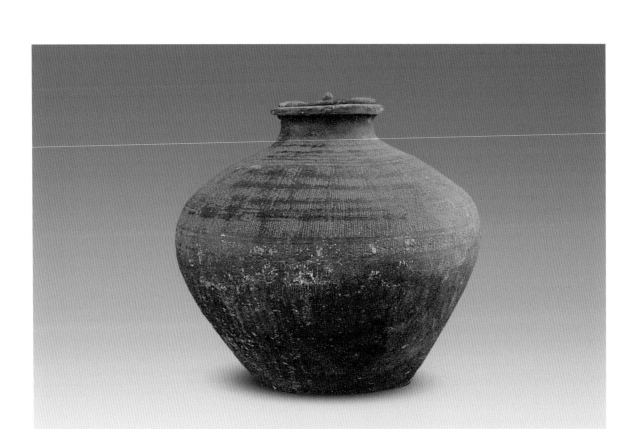

陶罐

汉

陶质

口径 11.5 厘米，底径 16.2 厘米，通高 27.8 厘米，重 3900 克

Pottery Jar

Han Dynasty

Pottery

Mouth Diameter 11.5 cm/ Bottom Diameter 16.2 cm/ Height 27.8 cm/ Weight 3,900 g

敞口，鼓腹，平底，周身绳纹，肩部有铭文。
完整无损。容器。陕西省渭南市澄城县征集。

陕西医史博物馆藏

This pottery jar has a flaring mouth, a rounded
body and a flat bottom. The whole jar is adorned
with cord patterns, with an inscription on the
shoulder. It served as a container and remains
intact. The jar was collected from Chengcheng
County of Weinan City, Shaanxi Province.
Preserved in Shaanxi Museum of Medical History

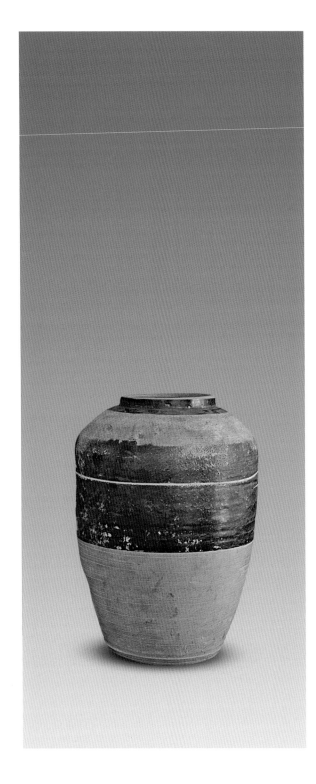

黑釉陶罐

汉

陶质

口径 11.5 厘米，底径 13.5 厘米，通高 29 厘米，

重 2600 克

Black-glazed Pottery Jar

Han Dynasty

Pottery

Mouth Diameter 11.5 cm/ Bottom Diameter 13.5 cm /

Height 29 cm/ weight 2,600 g

直口，折肩，斜腹，肩部无釉，腹 1/2 处无釉。
完整无损。盛贮器，生活用器具。

陕西医史博物馆藏

The jar features a straight mouth, a slightly
sloping shoulder, and a slightly tapering body.
The shoulder and the lower half of the belly are
unglazed. It served as a household container,
and remains intact.

Preserved in Shaanxi Museum of Medical History

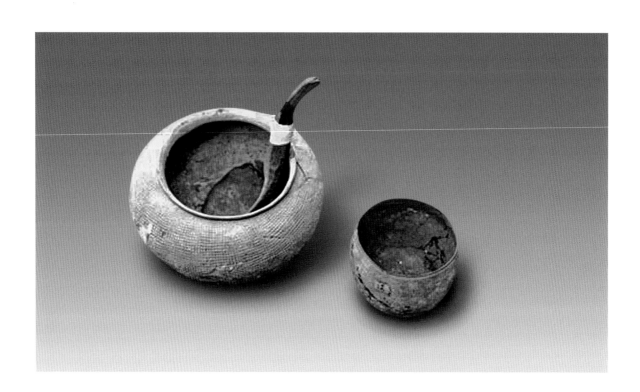

麻布纹罐一套

汉

陶质

大罐：上口直径 10.5 厘米，底部直径 8.2 厘米，罐身直径 16 厘米，腹深 9 厘米，最高 9.7 厘米

小罐：上口直径 7.6 厘米，底部直径 6 厘米，罐身直径 9.2 厘米，腹深 6.2 厘米，高 6.7 厘米

Set of Jars with Linen Patterns

Han Dynasty

Pottery

The big one: Mouth Diameter 10.5 cm/ Bottom Diameter 8.2 cm/ Belly Diameter 16 cm/ Depth 9 cm/ Height 9.7 cm

The small one: Mouth Diameter 7.6 cm/ Bottom Diameter 6 cm/ Belly Diameter 9.2 cm/ Depth 6.2 cm/ Height 6.7 cm

大罐：鼓腹，麻布纹，大口，侈唇外翻，平底。
储容器。

小罐：麻布纹，圆形，大口。储容器。

广东中医药博物馆藏

The big one: The jar has a wide mouth with an everted rim, a compressed globular body and a flat bottom. Its belly is adorned with linen patterns. The jar was used as a storage vessel.

The small one: The jar, covered with linen patterns, is a round vessel with a wide mouth. The jar was used as a storage vessel.

Preserved in Guangdong Chinese Medicine Museum

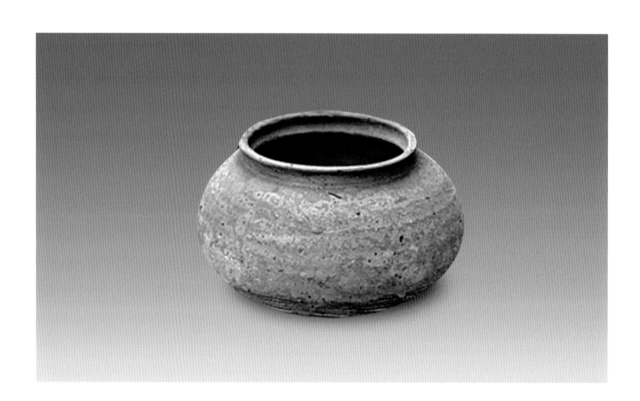

绳纹陶罐

汉

陶质

口外径 18.6 厘米，直径 30.5 厘米，腹深 17 厘米，通高 19.4 厘米

Pottery Jar with Cord Patterns

Han Dynasty

Pottery

Mouth Diameter 18.6 cm/ Diameter 30.5 cm/ Depth 17cm/ Height 19.4 cm

绳纹，敛口，侈唇外翻，鼓腹。储容器。

广东中医药博物馆藏

The jar, decorated with cord patterns, has a contracted mouth with its rim everted, and a compressed globular body. The jar was used as a storage vessel.

Preserved in Guangdong Chinese Medicine Museum

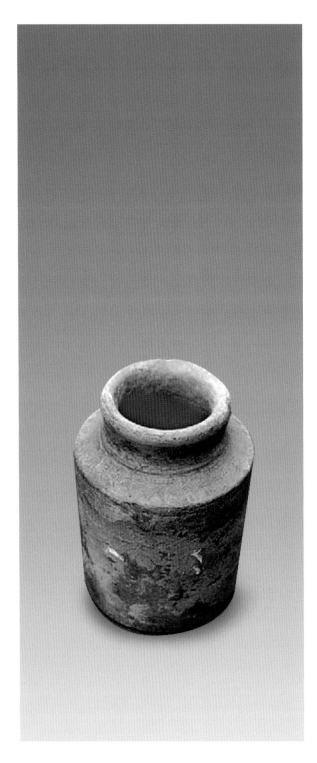

陶罐

汉

陶质

上口直径 6 厘米，底径 10 厘米，腹深 14 厘米，

高 18.3 厘米

圆柱形，大口，侈口稍外翻。储容器。

广东中医药博物馆藏

Pottery Jar

Han Dynasty

Pottery

Mouth Diameter 6 cm/ Bottom Diameter 10 cm/

Depth 14 cm/ Height 18.3 cm

The cylindrical jar has a wide mouth, with its rim

slightly everted. It was used as a storage vessel.

Preserved in Guangdong Chinese Medicine Museum

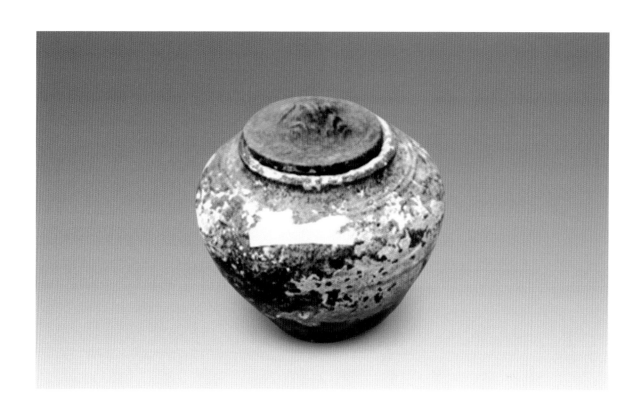

绿釉陶盖罐

汉

陶质

口外径 9.2 厘米，底径 7.5 厘米，腹径 15.0 厘米，

腹深 11.5 厘米，通高 14.3 厘米

带盖，敛口，鼓腹，圆圈底。盛物器。

广东中医药博物馆藏

Green-glazed Pottery Jar with Cover

Han Dynasty

Pottery

Mouth Diameter 9.2 cm/ Bottom Diameter 7.5 cm/
Belly Diameter 15.0 cm/ Depth 11.5 cm/ Height
14.3 cm

The jar, with a lid on the top, has a contracted
mouth, a globular body and a ring foot. It served as
a storage container.

Preserved in Guangdong Chinese Medicine Museum

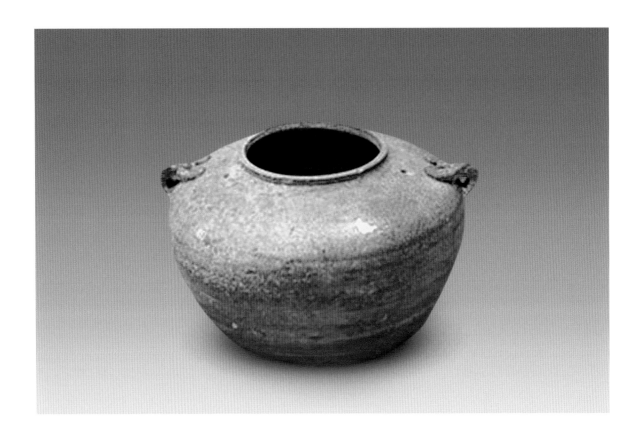

二系带釉陶罐

汉

陶质

口外径 10.9 厘米，底径 13.3 厘米，腹径 24 厘米，腹深 13.0 厘米，通高 14.5 厘米

Glazed Pottery Jar with Two Rings

Han Dynasty

Pottery

Mouth Diameter 10.9 cm/ Bottom Diameter 13.3 cm/ Belly Diameter 24 cm/ Depth 13cm/ Height 14.5 cm

绳纹，敛口，侈唇外翻，鼓腹。储容器。

广东中医药博物馆藏

The jar has a globular body covered with cord patterns, and a contracted mouth with its rim everted. The jar was used as a storage vessel. Preserved in Guangdong Chinese Medicine Museum

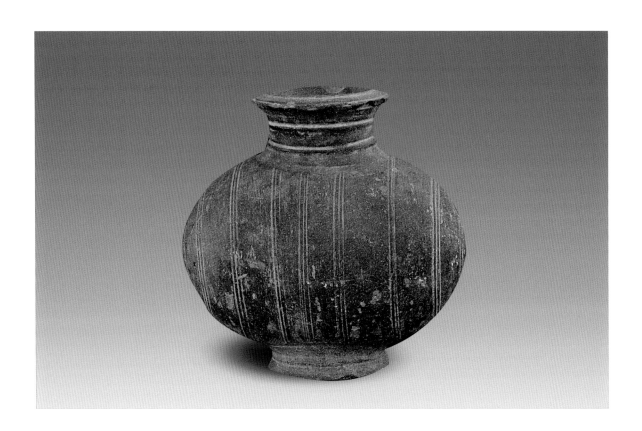

茧形陶壶

汉

灰陶质

口径 10 厘米，底径 9 厘米，通高 20.5 厘米，重 1300 克

Cocoon-shaped Pottery Pot

Han Dynasty

Grey Pottery

Mouth Diameter 10 cm/ Bottom Diameter 9 cm/ Height 20.5 cm/ Weight 1,300 g

喇叭形口沿，腹为椭圈形，圈足，颈部和腹部有弦纹。完整无损。容器。

陕西医史博物馆藏

The pot features a mouth in the shape of a trumpet, an oblong body and a ring foot. String patterns can be seen around its neck and belly. The well-preserved pot served as a container.

Preserved in Shaanxi Museum of Medical History

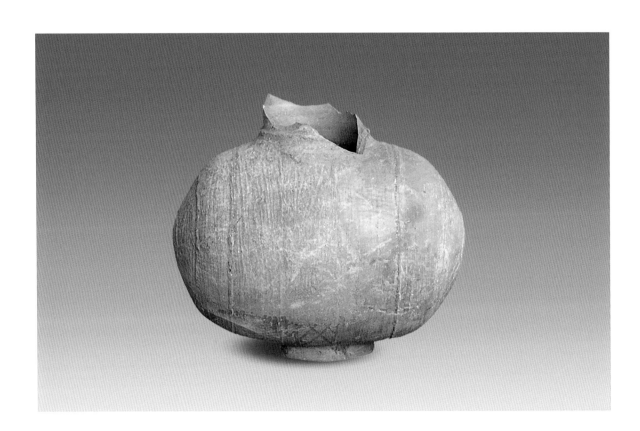

茧形壶

汉

陶质

底径 7 厘米，重 1050 克

Cocoon-shaped Pot

Han Dynasty

Pottery

Bottom Diameter 7 cm/ Weight 1,050 g

腹为茧形，浅圈足，腹有八道环形纹，灰陶。

口颈全残。生活器具。陕西省澄城县征集。

陕西医史博物馆藏

The pot is made of grey pottery with a cocoon-shaped belly which is decorated with eight vertical bands of patterns. It has a shallow ring foot. Its mouth and neck are damaged completely. The pot was used as a household utensil, and was collected from Chengcheng County, Shaanxi Province.

Preserved in Shaanxi Museum of Medical History

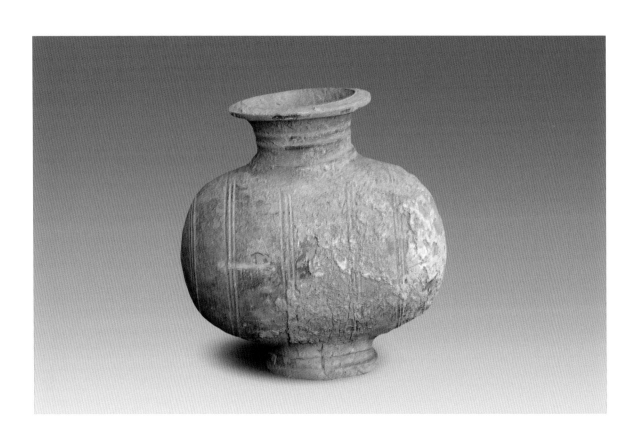

茧形壶

汉

陶质

口径 11 厘米，底径 9 厘米，高 20 厘米，重 1500 克

Cocoon-shaped Pot

Han Dynasty

Pottery

Mouth Diameter 11 cm/ Bottom Diameter 9 cm/ Height 20 cm/ Weight 1,500 g

平口沿，侈口，短颈，茧形腹，圈足，圈足
上有一印记，颈有三道弦纹，腹部八道环形
纹，灰陶。生活器具。陕西省白水县杨家沟
征集。

陕西医史博物馆藏

The grey pottery pot features a flat mouth rim,
a flared mouth, a short neck, a cocoon-shaped
belly and a ring foot. A seal can be seen on
its ring foot. Three rings of string patterns are
carved on the neck of the pot and eight bands of
vertical patterns on its belly. The pot was used
as a household utensil and was collected from
Yangjiagou, Baishui County, Shaanxi Province.
Preserved in Shaanxi Museum of Medical History

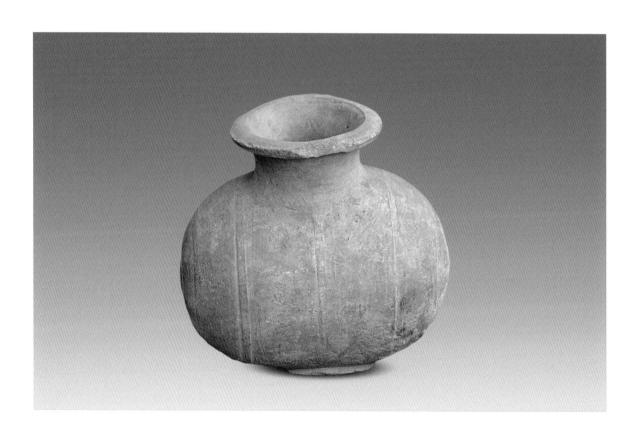

茧形壶

汉

陶质

口径 10.05 厘米，底径 8 厘米，高 5.4 厘米，重 1200 克

Cocoon-shaped Pot

Han Dynasty

Pottery

Mouth Diameter 10.05 cm/ Bottom Diameter 8 cm/ Height 5.4 cm/ Weight 1,200 g

平口沿，侈口，短颈，茧形腹，浅圈足，腹部七道环形纹，灰陶，陶质较粗。口沿略残。生活器具。陕西省白水县征集。

陕西医史博物馆收藏

This grey pottery pot, a piece of coarse grey pottery, has a flat mouth rim, a flared mouth, a short neck, a cocoon-shaped belly and a shallow ring foot. Its belly is incised with seven bands of vertical patterns. The pot was used as a household utensil and its mouth rim was slightly damaged. It was collected from Baishui County, Shaanxi Province.

Preserved in Shaanxi Museum of Medical History

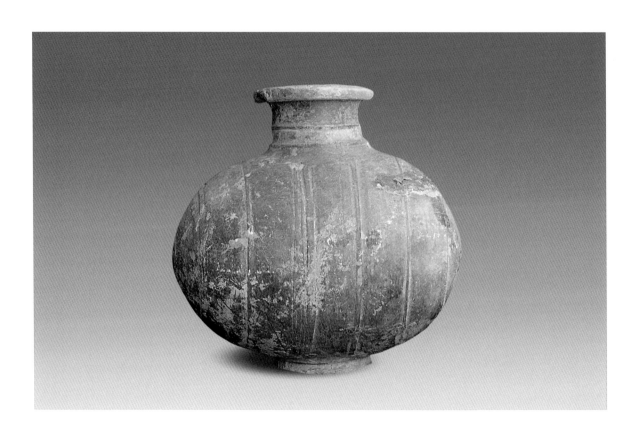

茧形壶

汉

陶质

口径 10 厘米，底径 8.5 厘米，高 22.8 厘米，重 1900 克

Cocoon-shaped Pot

Han Dynasty

Pottery

Mouth Diameter 10 cm/ Bottom Diameter 8.5 cm/ Height 22.8 cm/ Weight 1,900 g

平口沿，短颈，腹为茧形，圈足，腹部有八
道环形纹，灰陶。完整无损。生活器具。陕
西省澄城县征集。

陕西医史博物馆藏

The grey pottery pot has a flat mouth rim, a
short neck, a cocoon-shaped belly and a ring
foot. Eight bands of vertical patterns are carved
on its belly. The pot was used as a household
utensil and remains intact. It was collected from
Chengcheng County, Shaanxi Province.

Preserved in Shaanxi Museum of Medical History

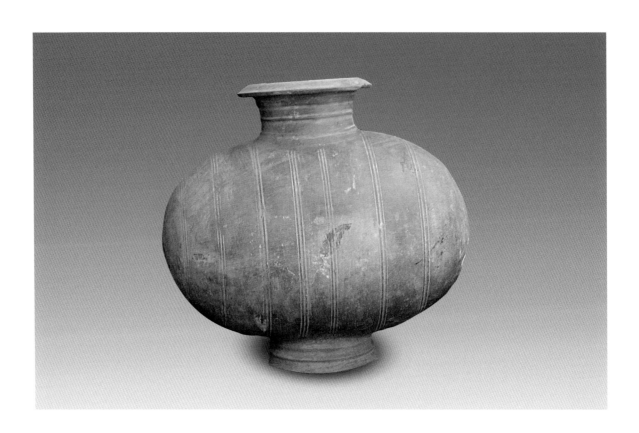

茧形壶

汉

陶质

口径 12.5 厘米，底径 10.6 厘米，高 25.6 厘米，重 2000 克

Cocoon-shaped Pot

Han Dynasty

Pottery

Mouth Diameter 12.5 cm/ Bottom Diameter 10.6 cm/ Height 25.6 cm/ Weight 2,000 g

侈口，口沿外翻，短颈，腹为茧形，圈足，
腹部有十道环形纹，灰陶。口沿残。生活器具。
陕西省澄城县征集。

陕西医史博物馆藏

The grey pottery pot has a flared mouth with
an everted mouth rim, a short neck, a cocoon-
shaped belly and a ring foot. Ten bands of
vertical patterns can be seen on its belly. Its
mouth rim is damaged. The pot was used as a
household utensil, and pot was collected from
Chengcheng County, Shaanxi Province.
Preserved in Shaanxi Museum of Medical History

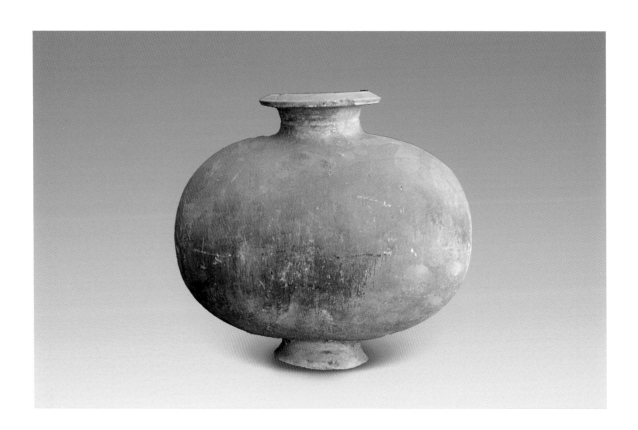

茧形壶

汉

陶质

口径 12.5 厘米，底径 10 厘米，高 27 厘米，重 2350 克

Cocoon-shaped Pot

Han Dynasty

Pottery

Mouth Diameter 12.5 cm/ Bottom Diameter 10 cm/ Height 27 cm/ Weight 2,350 g

口沿外翻，侈口，短颈，茧形腹，圈足。完
整无损。生活器具。陕西省澄城县征集。

陕西医史博物馆藏

The pot has an everted mouth rim, a flared
mouth, a short neck, a cocoon-shaped belly and
a ring foot. The pot was used as a household
utensil and has been preserved intact, and was
collected from Chengcheng County, Shaanxi
Province.

Preserved in Shaanxi Museum of Medical History

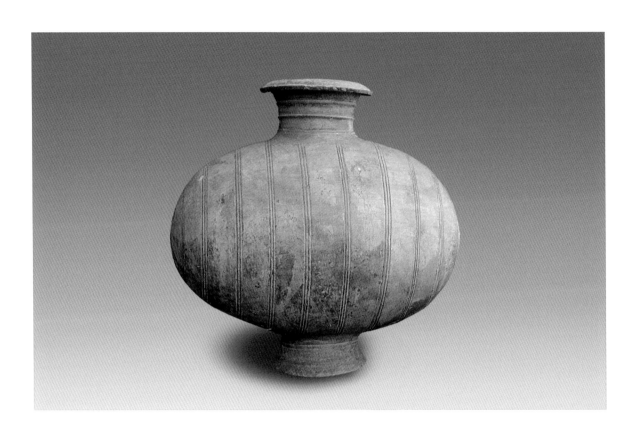

茧形壶

汉

陶质

口径 13.5 厘米，底径 12.2 厘米，高 34.5 厘米，重 3050 克

Cocoon-shaped Pot

Han Dynasty

Pottery

Mouth Diameter 13.5 cm/ Bottom Diameter 12.2 cm/ Height 34.5 cm/ Weight 3,050 g

口沿外翻，侈口，短颈，茧形腹，高圈足，腹部有十二道环形纹，灰陶。口沿残。生活器具。陕西省澄城县征集。

陕西医史博物馆藏

The grey pottery pot has an everted mouth rim, a flared mouth, a short neck, a cocoon-shaped belly and a high ring foot. Its belly is decorated with twelve bands of vertical patterns. Its mouth rim is damaged. The pot was used as a household utensil, and was collected from Chengcheng County, Shaanxi Province.

Preserved in Shaanxi Museum of Medical History

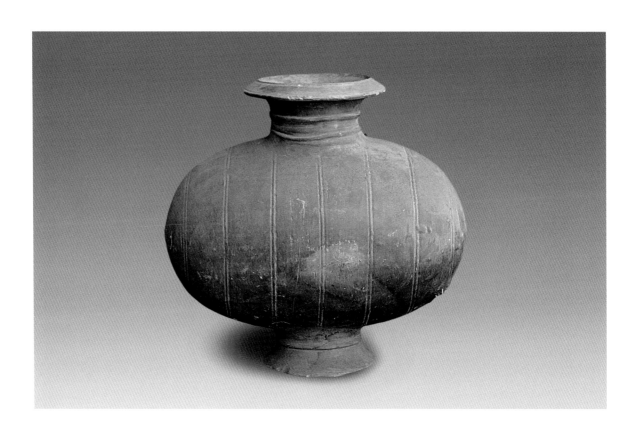

茧形壶

汉

陶质

口径 12 厘米，底径 10.5 厘米，高 24.7 厘米，重 1750 克

Cocoon-shaped Pot

Han Dynasty

Pottery

Mouth Diameter 12 cm/ Bottom Diameter 10.5 cm/ Height 24.7 cm/ Weight 1,750 g

口沿外翻，侈口，短颈，茧形腹，倒喇叭底，腹部九道环形纹，灰陶。口沿残。生活器具。陕西省澄城县征集。

陕西医史博物馆收藏

The grey pottery pot has an everted mouth rim, a flared mouth, a short neck, a cocoon-shaped belly and an inverted trumpet-shaped bottom. Its belly is decorated with nine bands of vertical patterns. The meth rim is damaged. The pot was used as a household utensil, and was collected from Chengcheng County, Shaanxi Province. Preserved in Shaanxi Museum of Medical History

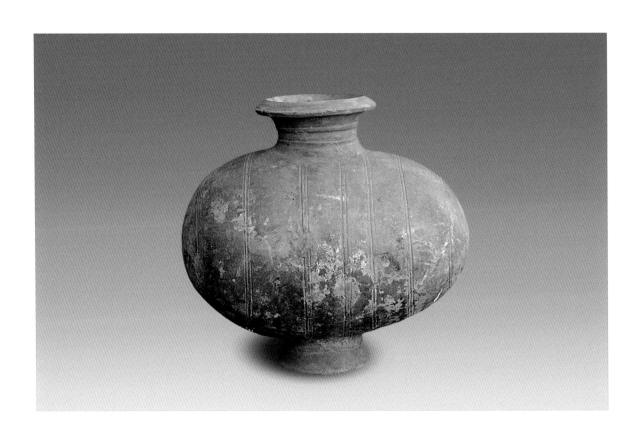

茧形壶

汉

陶质

口径 11.5 厘米，底径 9.2 厘米，高 24.5 厘米，重 1750 克

Cocoon-shaped Pot

Han Dynasty

Pottery

Mouth Diameter 11.5 cm/ Bottom Diameter 9.2 cm/ Height 24.5 cm/ Weight 1,750 g

口沿外翻，侈口，短颈，茧形腹，腹部有九道环形纹，圈足。完整无损。生活器具。陕西省澄城县征集。

陕西医史博物馆收藏

The pot has an everted mouth rim, a flared mouth, a short neck, a cocoon-shaped belly and a ring foot. Its belly is decorated with nine bands of vertical patterns. The pot was used as a household utensil and has been preserved well. It was collected from Chengcheng County, Shaanxi Province.

Preserved in Shaanxi Museum of Medical History

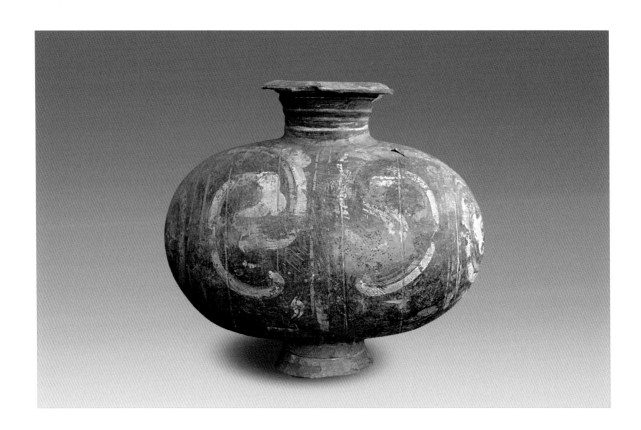

茧形壶

汉

陶质

口径 13 厘米，底径 10 厘米，高 27 厘米，重 2400 克

Cocoon-shaped Pot

Han Dynasty

Pottery

Mouth Diameter 13 cm/ Bottom Diameter 10 cm/ Height 27 cm/ Weight 2,400 g

口沿外翻，侈口，短颈，茧形腹，圈足，腹部有八道环形纹，通身施有彩绘，灰陶。口沿、底略残，肩有一小孔。生活器具。陕西省白水县征集。

陕西医史博物馆藏

The grey pottery pot has an everted mouth rim, a flared mouth, a short neck, a cocoon-shaped belly and a ring foot. Its belly is decorated with eight vertical bands of patterns and its whole body with coloured drawings. Its mouth rim and bottom are slightly damaged. A small hole can be found on its shoulder. The pot was used as a household utensil, and was collected from Baishui County, Shaanxi Province.

Preserved in Shaanxi Museum of Medical History

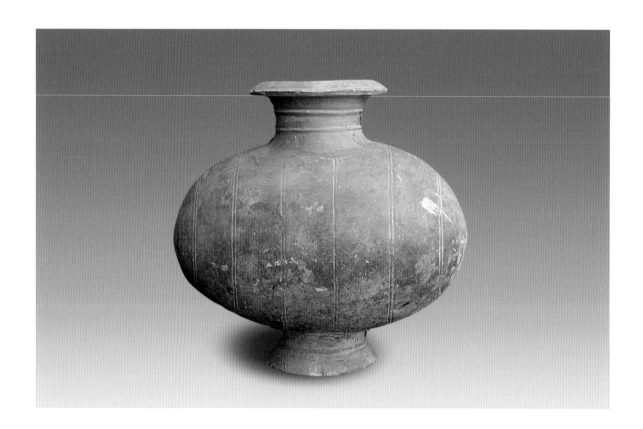

茧形壶

汉

陶质

口径 12.5 厘米，底径 10.1 厘米，高 24.2 厘米，重 1600 克

Cocoon-shaped Pot

Han Dynasty

Pottery

Mouth Diameter 12.5 cm/ Bottom Diameter 10.1 cm/ Height 24.2 cm/ Weight 1,600 g

口沿外翻，侈口，短颈，茧形腹，倒喇叭底，
腹部有八道环形纹，灰陶。口沿、底略残。
生活器具。陕西省澄城县征集。

陕西医史博物馆藏

The grey pottery pot has an everted mouth rim, a flared mouth, a short neck, a cocoon-shaped belly and an inverted trumpet-shaped bottom. Eight bands of vertical patterns can be seen on its belly. Its mouth rim and bottom are slightly damaged. The pot was used as a household utensil, and was collected from Chengcheng County, Shaanxi Province.

Preserved in Shaanxi Museum of Medical History

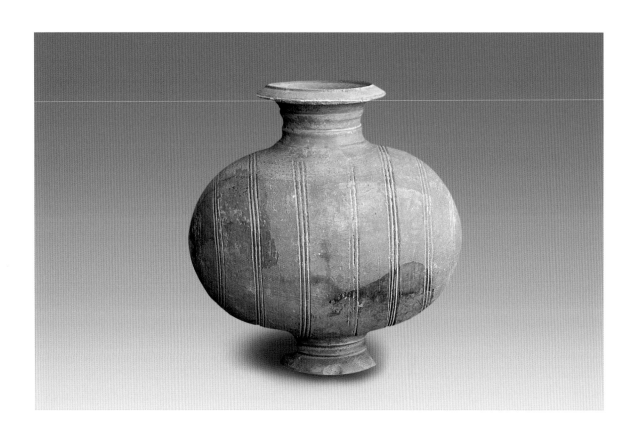

茧形壶

汉

陶质

口径 12 厘米，底径 9.9 厘米，高 25.1 厘米，重 1600 克

Cocoon-shaped Pot

Han Dynasty

Pottery

Mouth Diameter 12 cm/ Bottom Diameter 9.9 cm/ Height 25.1 cm/ Weight 1,600 g

口沿外翻，侈口，短颈，茧形腹，圈足，腹部有十道环形纹，底座有二道凸棱。底残。生活器具。陕西省澄城县征集。

陕西医史博物馆收藏

The pot has an everted mouth rim, a flared mouth, a short neck, a cocoon-shaped belly and a ring foot. On its belly are carved ten bands of vertical patterns, and the bottom, slightly damaged, is decorated with two rings of raised ridges. The pot was used as a household utensil, and was collected from Chengcheng County, Shaanxi Province.

Preserved in Shaanxi Museum of Medical History

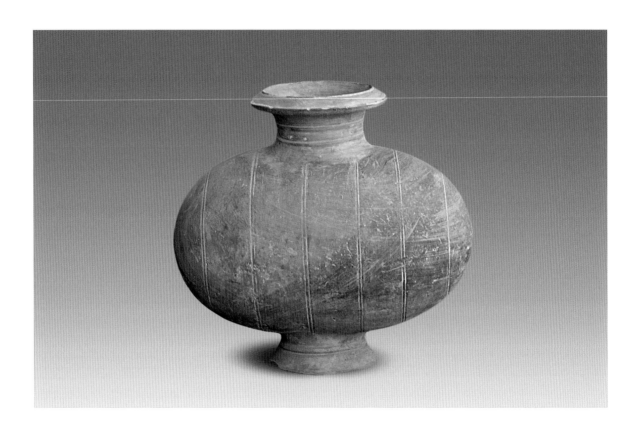

茧形壶

汉

陶质

口径 12 厘米，底径 3.5 厘米，高 9.5 厘米，重 1700 克

Cocoon-shaped Pot

Han Dynasty

Pottery

Mouth Diameter 12 cm/ Bottom Diameter 3.5 cm/ Height 9.5 cm/ Weight 1,700 g

口沿外翻，侈口，茧形腹，倒喇叭形底座，腹部有八道环形纹，灰陶。口沿和底略残。生活器具。陕西省澄城县征集。

陕西医史博物馆藏

The grey pottery pot has an everted mouth rim, a flared mouth, a cocoon-shaped belly and an inverted trumpet-shaped bottom. Eight bands of vertical patterns can be seen on its belly. Its mouth rim and bottom are slightly damaged. The pot was used as a household utensil, and was collected from Chengcheng County, Shaanxi Province.

Preserved in Shaanxi Museum of Medical History

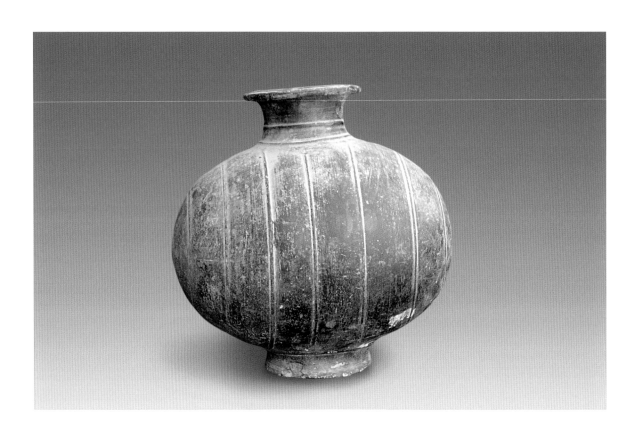

茧形壶

汉

陶质

口径 13.5 厘米，底径 12.6 厘米，高 30 厘米，重 3450 克

Cocoon-shaped Pot

Han Dynasty

Pottery

Mouth Diameter 13.5 cm/ Bottom Diameter 12.6 cm/ Height 30 cm/ Weight 3,450 g

平口沿，侈口，短颈，茧形腹，圈足，腹部有九道环形纹，灰陶。口沿和底略残。生活器具。陕西省澄城县征集。

陕西医史博物馆藏

The grey pottery pot has a flat mouth rim, a flared mouth, a short neck, a cocoon-shaped belly and a ring foot. Nine bands of vertical patterns can be seen on its belly. Its mouth rim and bottom are slightly damaged. The pot was used as a household utensil, and was collected from Chengcheng County, Shaanxi Province.

Preserved in Shaanxi Museum of Medical History

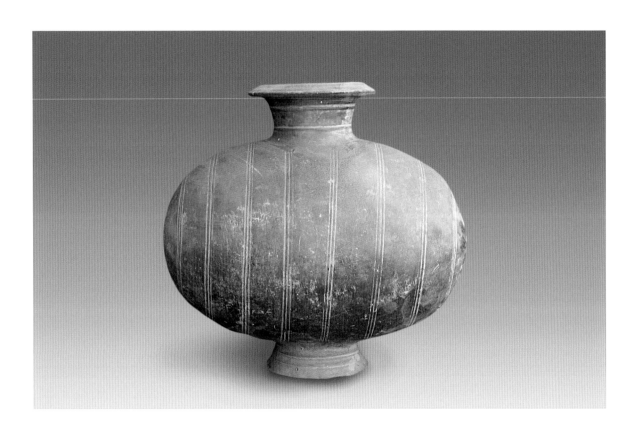

茧形壶

汉

陶质

口径 14 厘米，底径 11.5 厘米，高 30 厘米

Cocoon-shaped Pot

Han Dynasty

Pottery

Mouth Diameter 14 cm/ Bottom Diameter 11.5 cm/ Height 30 cm

口沿外翻，侈口，短颈，茧形腹，腹部有十
道环形纹，灰陶。口沿残。生活器具。陕西
省澄城县征集。

陕西医史博物馆藏

The grey pottery pot has an everted mouth
rim, a flared mouth, a short neck and a cocoon-
shaped belly. Ten bands of vertical patterns can
be seen on its belly. Its mouth rim is damaged.
The pot was used as a household utensil,
and was collected from Chengcheng County,
Shaanxi Province.

Preserved in Shaanxi Museum of Medical History

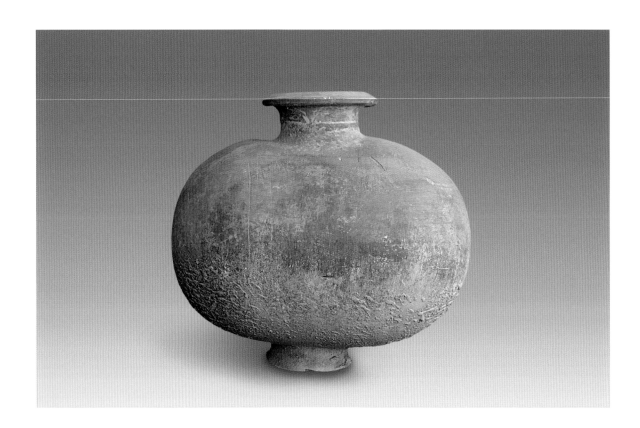

茧形壶

汉

陶质

口径 12 厘米，底径 9 厘米，高 27.5 厘米

Cocoon-shaped Pot

Han Dynasty

Pottery

Mouth Diameter 12 cm/ Bottom Diameter 9 cm/ Height 27.5 cm

口沿外翻，侈口，短颈，茧形腹，圈足，素面，灰陶。完整无损。生活器具。陕西省澄城县征集。

陕西医史博物馆藏

The grey pot, with no decoration, has an everted mouth rim, a flared mouth, a short neck, a cocoon-shaped belly and a ring foot. The pot was used as a household utensil and remains intact. It was collected from Chengcheng County, Shaanxi Province.

Preserved in Shaanxi Museum of Medical History

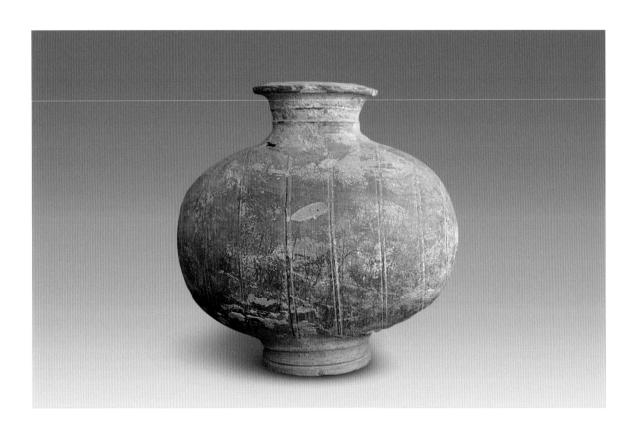

茧形壶

汉

陶质

口径 12 厘米，底径 11 厘米，高 5.4 厘米，重 2500 克

Cocoon-shaped Pot

Han Dynasty

Pottery

Mouth Diameter 12 cm/ Bottom Diameter 11 cm/ Height 5.4 cm/ Weight 2,500 g

平口沿，侈口，短颈，茧形腹，圈足，圈足
上有一印记，腹部有十道环形纹，灰陶。生
活器具。陕西省澄城县征集。

陕西医史博物馆藏

The grey pot features with a flat mouth rim, a
flared mouth, a short neck, a cocoon-shaped
belly and a ring foot on which a seal can be
seen. Its belly is decorated with ten bands
of vertical patterns. The pot was used as a
household utensil, and was collected from
Chengcheng County, Shaanxi Province.

Preserved in Shaanxi Museum of Medical History

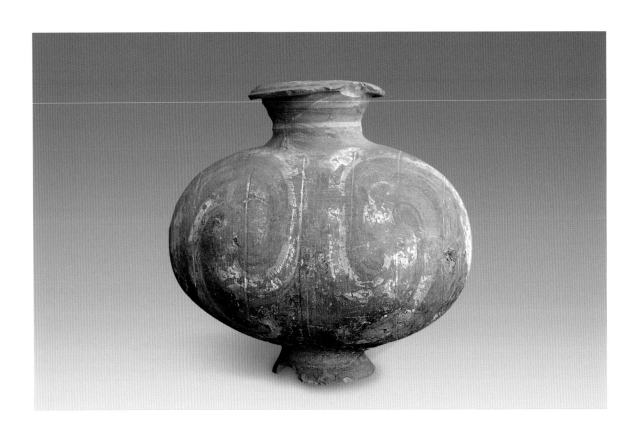

茧形壶

汉

陶质

口径 11 厘米，底径 9 厘米，高 23.5 厘米，重 1650 克

Cocoon-shaped Pot

Han Dynasty

Pottery

Mouth Diameter 11 cm/ Bottom Diameter 9 cm/ Height 23.5 cm/ Weight 1,650 g

口沿外翻，侈口，短颈，茧形腹，圈足，腹
部有八道环形纹，并饰有彩绘，灰陶。口、腹、
底都有残。生活器具。陕西省水白县征集。

陕西医史博物馆藏

The prey pottery pot has a flared mouth with
an everted mouth rim, a short neck, a cocoon-
shaped belly and a ring foot. Its belly is
decorated with eight bands of vertical patterns
and coloured drawings. Its mouth rim, belly
and bottom are damaged to different degrees.
The pot was used as a household utensil, and
was collected from Baishui County, Shaanxi
Province.

Preserved in Shaanxi Museum of Medical History

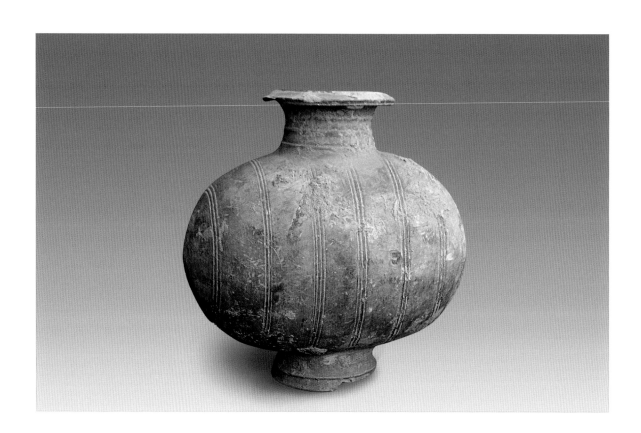

茧形壶

汉

陶质

口径 11.5 厘米，底径 10 厘米，高 23.5 厘米，重 1800 克

Cocoon-shaped Pot

Han Dynasty

Pottery

Mouth Diameter 11.5 cm/ Bottom Diameter 10 cm/ Height 23.5 cm/ Weight 1,800 g

口沿外翻，侈口，短颈，茧形壶，圈足，腹
部有九道弦纹，灰陶。口沿和底都残。生活
器具。陕西省澄城县征集。

陕西医史博物馆藏

The grey pottery pot has a flared mouth with
an everted mouth rim, a short neck, a cocoon-
shaped belly and a ring foot. Nine vertical bands
of decorations can be seen on its belly.Its mouth
rim and bottom are damaged. The pot was used
as a household utensil, and was collected from
Chengcheng County, Shaanxi Province.

Preserved in Shaanxi Museum of Medical History

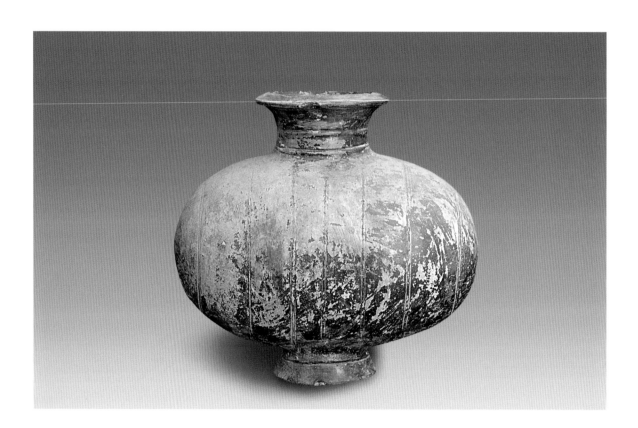

茧形壶

汉

陶质

口径 12.5 厘米，底径 9.8 厘米，高 25.5 厘米，重 1650 克

Cocoon-shaped Pot

Han Dynasty

Pottery

Mouth Diameter 12.5 cm/ Bottom Diameter 9.8 cm/ Height 25.5 cm/ Weight 1,650 g

侈口，口沿外翻，短颈，腹为茧形，圈足，腹部有七道环形纹，灰陶。口沿略残。生活器具。陕西省澄城县征集。

陕西医史博物馆藏

The grey pottery pot has a flared mouth with an everted mouth rim, a short neck, a cocoon-shaped belly and a ring foot. Its belly is incised with seven bands of vertical patterns. Its mouth rim is slightly damaged. The pot was used as a household utensil, and was collected from Chengcheng County, Shaanxi Province.

Preserved in Shaanxi Museum of Medical History

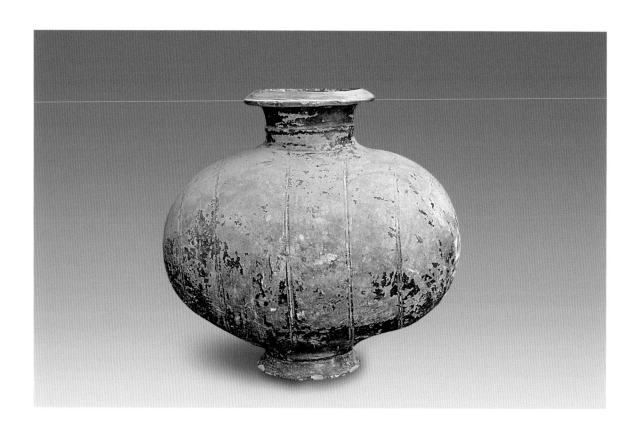

茧形壶

汉

陶质

口径 12 厘米，底径 9.5 厘米，高 23.5 厘米，重 1700 克

Cocoon-shaped Pot

Han Dynasty

Pottery

Mouth Diameter 12 cm/ Bottom Diameter 9.5 cm/ Height 23.5 cm/ Weight 1,700 g

侈口，口沿外翻，短颈，腹为茧形，圈足，腹部有六道环形纹，灰陶。完整无损。生活器具。陕西省澄城县征集。

陕西医史博物馆藏

The grey pottery pot has a flared mouth with an everted mouth rim, a short neck, a cocoon-shaped belly and a ring foot. Its belly is decorated with six bands of vertical patterns. The pot was used as a household utensil and has been preserved well. It was collected from Chengcheng County, Shaanxi Province.

Preserved in Shaanxi Museum of Medical History

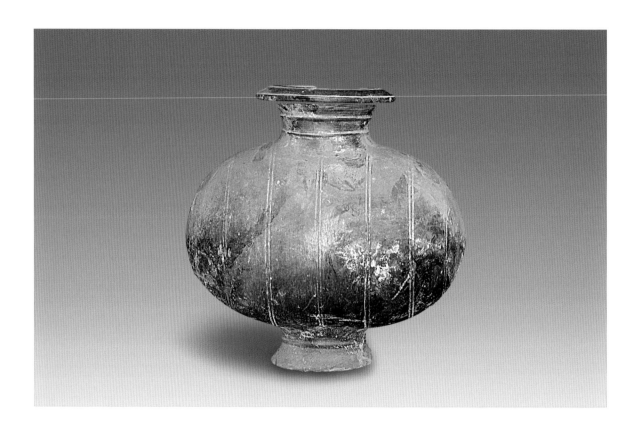

茧形壶

汉

陶质

口径 12 厘米，底径 9.8 厘米，高 22.8 厘米，重 1750 克

Cocoon-shaped Pot

Han Dynasty

Pottery

Mouth Diameter 12 cm/ Bottom Diameter 9.8 cm/ Height 22.8 cm/ Weight 1,750 g

口沿外翻，侈口，短颈，茧形腹，腹有九道
环形纹，圈足，灰陶。口沿残，底略残。生
活器具。陕西省澄城县征集。

陕西医史博物馆藏

The grey pottery pot has a flared mouth with
an everted mouth rim, a short neck, a cocoon-
shaped belly and a ring foot. Nine bands of
vertical patterns can be seen on its belly. Its
mouth rim and bottom are damaged to different
degrees. The pot was used as a household
utensil, and was collected from Chengcheng
County, Shaanxi Province.

Preserved in Shaanxi Museum of Medical History

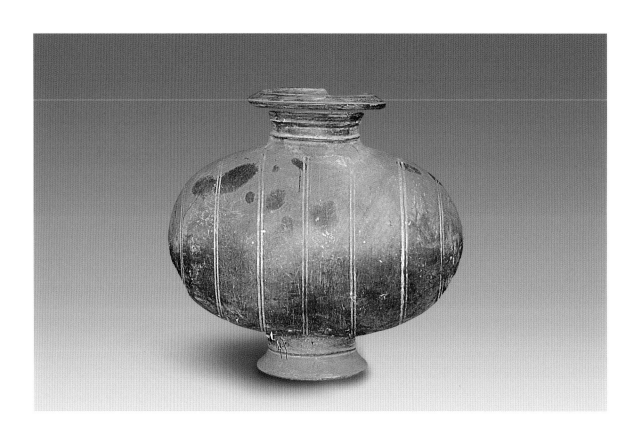

茧形壶

汉

陶质

口径 12.5 厘米，底径 10 厘米，高 24 厘米，重 1700 克

Cocoon-shaped Pot

Han Dynasty

Pottery

Mouth Diameter 12.5 cm/ Bottom Diameter 10 cm/ Height 24 cm/ Weight 1,700 g

口沿外翻，侈口，短颈，茧形腹，圈足腹部
有九道环形纹，灰陶。口残。生活器具。陕
西省澄城县征集。

陕西医史博物馆藏

The grey pottery pot has a flared mouth with
an everted mouth rim, a short neck, a cocoon-
shaped belly and a ring foot. Nine vertical
bands of decorations can be seen on its belly.
Its mouth rim is damaged. The pot was used
as a household utensil, and was collected from
Chengcheng County, Shaanxi Province.
Preserved in Shaanxi Museum of Medical History

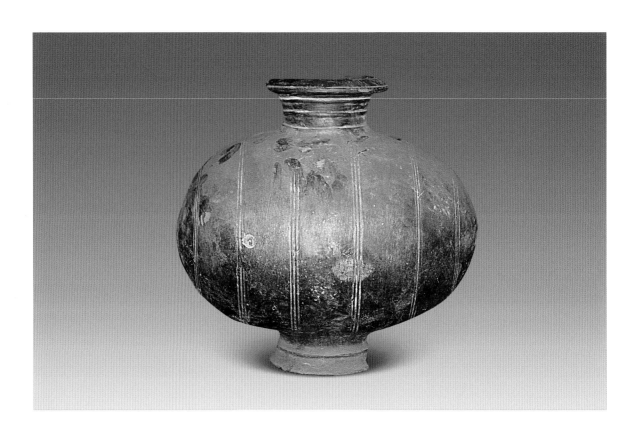

茧形壶

汉

陶质

口径 11.5 厘米，底径 10 厘米，高 24.9 厘米，重 2000 克

Cocoon-shaped Pot

Han Dynasty

Pottery

Mouth Diameter 11.5 cm/ Bottom Diameter 10 cm/ Height 24.9 cm/ Weight 2,000 g

口沿外翻，短颈，茧形腹，圈足，腹部有八
道环形纹，灰陶。口底残。生活器具。陕西
省澄城县征集。

陕西医史博物馆藏

The grey pottery pot has a flared mouth with
an everted mouth rim, a short neck, a cocoon-
shaped belly and a ring foot. Eight bands of
vertical strings are carved on its body. Its mouth
and bottom are damaged. The pot served as
a household utensil, and was collected from
Chengcheng county, shaanxi Province.

Preserved in Shaanxi Museum of Medical History

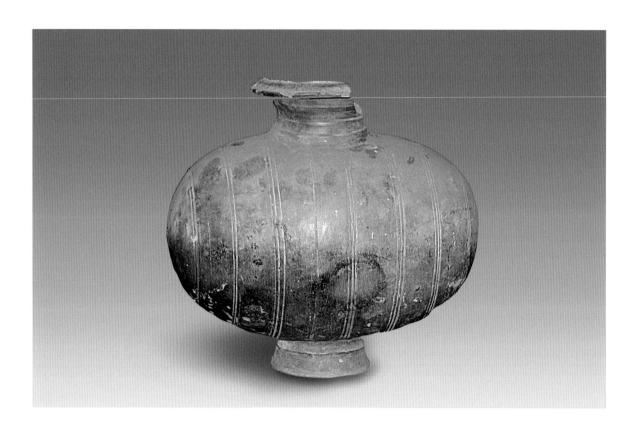

茧形壶

汉

陶质

口径 11.5 厘米，底径 9 厘米，高 24.2 厘米，重 1850 克

Cocoon-shaped Pot

Han Dynasty

Pottery

Mouth Diameter 11.5 cm/ Bottom Diameter 9 cm/ Height 24.2 cm/ Weight 1,850 g

□沿外翻，侈口，短颈，茧形腹，圈足，腹部有十道环形纹，灰陶。□残。生活器具。陕西省澄城县征集。

陕西医史博物馆藏

The grey pottery pot has a flared mouth with an everted mouth rim, a short neck, a cocoon-shaped belly and a ring foot. Ten bands of vertical strings are carved on its belly. Its mouth is damaged. The pot was used as a household utensil and was collected from Chengcheng County, Shaanxi Province.

Preserved in Shaanxi Museum of Medical History

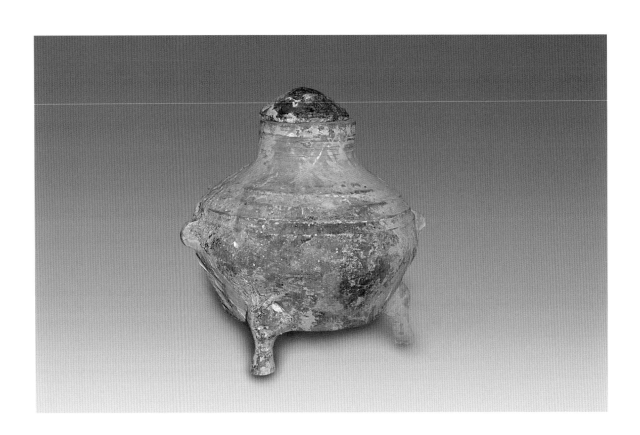

陶三足壶

汉

陶质

口径 6 厘米，底径 10.02 厘米，通高 17 厘米，足高 2.5 厘米，重 850 克

Tripod Pottery Pot

Han Dynasty

Grey pottery

Mouth Diameter 6 cm/ Bottom Diameter 10.02 cm/ Height 17 cm/ Height of The Foot 2.5 cm/ Weight 850 g

子母口，圆肩，平底，三蹄足，腹部有双耳，肩部三道弦纹，灰陶，带一蘑菇形盖。完整无损。生活器具。陕北征集。

陕西医史博物馆藏

This pot has a snap lid the shape of a mushroom, a rounded shoulder, a flat bottom, and three horseshoe-shaped feet. On its belly is a pair of handles, and on its shoulder are three circles of string patterns. The pot was used as a household utensil and remains intact. It was collected in Northern Shaanxi Province.

Preserved in Shaanxi Museum of Medical History

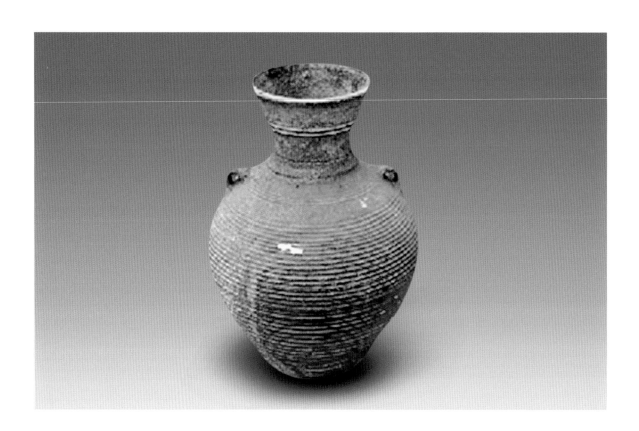

黄釉双系壶

汉

陶质

口外径 13.9 厘米， 底口径 12.8 厘米 ，腹径
25.4 厘米， 腹深 32.4 厘米，通高 34 厘米

鸭蛋形，双耳。储器。

广东中医药博物馆藏

Yellow-glazed Pot with Double Handles

Han Dynasty

Pottery

Outer Mouth Diameter13.9 cm/ Bottom Diameter
12.8 cm/ Belly Diameter 25.4 cm/ Depth 32.4 cm/
Height 34 cm

This double-handled pot is oval in shape. It was
used as a container.

Preserved in Guangdong Chinese Medicine Museum

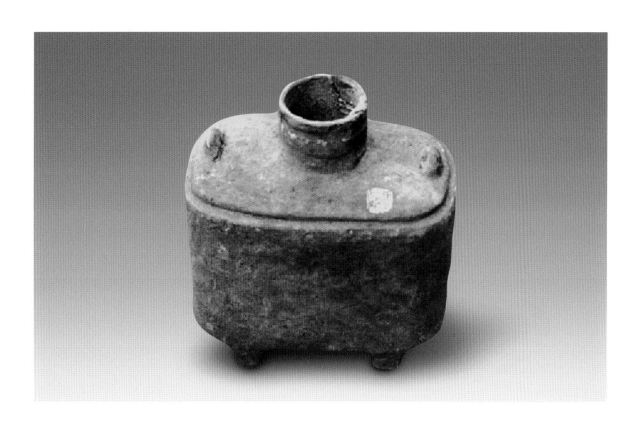

方形陶壶

汉

陶质

上口直径 2.4 厘米，壶身直径 11.1 厘米，壶深
12.6 厘米，底部长 11.5 厘米，底部宽 6.5 厘米，
高 15 厘米

长方形，方脚四只，小口。盛液体食物如水、酒
等的容器。

广东中医药博物馆藏

Squared Pottery Pot

Han Dynasty

Pottery

Mouth Diameter 2.4 cm/ Body Diameter 11.1 cm/
Depth 12.6 cm/ Bottom Length 11.5 cm/ Bottom
Width 6.5 cm/ Height 15 cm

This rectangular pot has four squared feet and a
narrow mouth. It was used as a water container or
wine vessel.

Preserved in Guangdong Chinese Medicine Museum

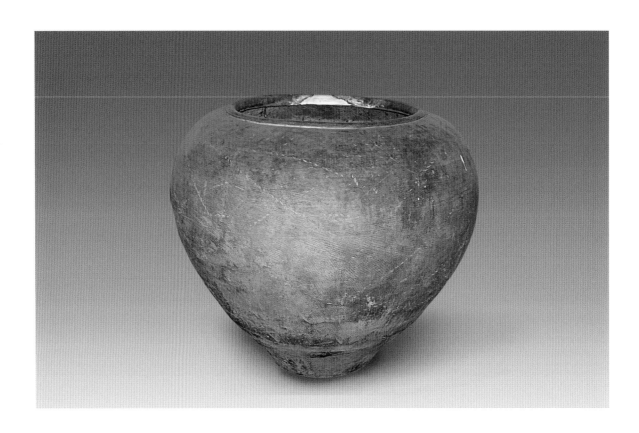

陶瓮

汉

灰陶质

口径 58 厘米，底径 28 厘米，通高 78 厘米

Pottery Urn

Han Dynasty

Grey Pottery

Mouth Diameter 58 cm/ Bottom Diameter 28 cm/ Height 78 cm

圆厚唇，鼓腹，平底，下腹部有绳纹和一指
纹饰。稍残，有修补。大型贮藏器具。陕西
省鄠邑区征集。

陕西医史博物馆藏

This pottery urn has a round and thick mouth
rim, a globular body and a flat bottom. The
lower part of its belly is decorated with cord
patterns and a fingerprint design. The urn is
slightly damaged and has been repaired. This
big container was collected in Huyi District,
Shaanxi Province.

Preserved in Shaanxi Museum of Medical History

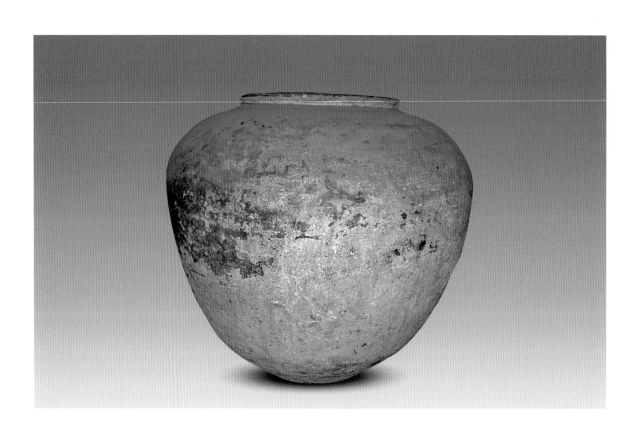

陶瓮

汉

灰陶质

口径 45.5 厘米，底径 24 厘米，通高 76 厘米

圆厚唇，圆肩，圆腹，平底，表面无纹饰。完整
无损。大型贮藏器具。陕西省长安区征集。

陕西医史博物馆藏

Pottery Urn

Han Dynasty

Grey Pottery

Mouth Diameter 45.5 cm/ Bottom Diameter 24 cm/
Height 76 cm

This pottery urn has a round and thick mouth rim,
a rounded shoulder, a globular body and a flat
bottom. There is no decoration on its surface. This
large container is still in perfect condition. It was
collected in Chang'an District, Shaanxi Province.
Preserved in Shaanxi Museum of Medical History

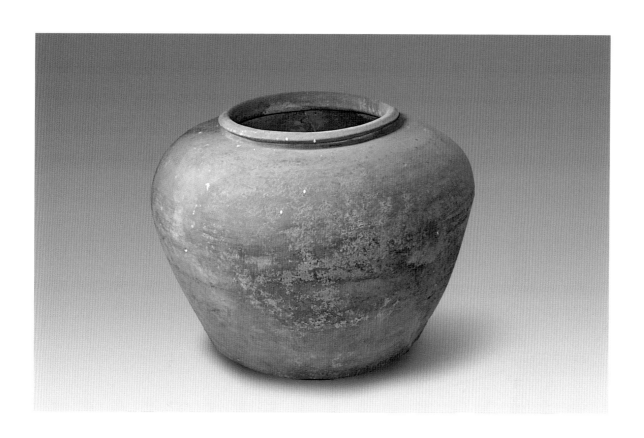

陶瓮

汉

灰陶质

口径 44 厘米，底径 23 厘米，通高 73 厘米

圆厚唇，平底，鼓腹，表面无纹饰。完整无损。

大型贮藏器具。陕西省咸阳市征集。

陕西医史博物馆藏

Pottery Urn

Han Dynasty

Grey Pottery

Mouth Diameter 44 cm/ Bottom Diameter 23 cm/
Height 73 cm

This pottery urn, a large container with no decoration,
has a round and thick mouth rim, a globular body and
a flat bottom. It remains intact and was collected in
Xianyang City, Shaanxi Province.

Preserved in Shaanxi Museum of Medical History

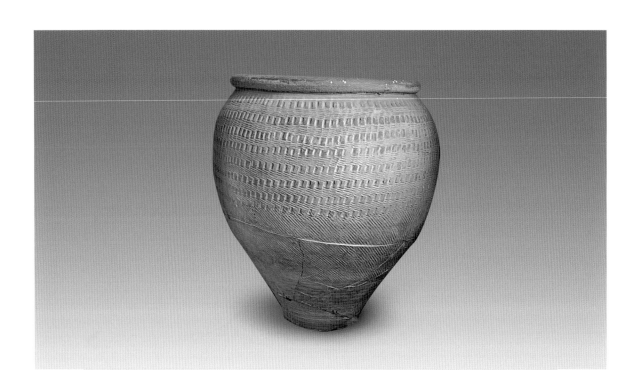

陶瓮

汉

陶质

口径 66 厘米，底径 28 厘米，通高 95 厘米

厚圆唇，圆腹，平底，上腹短而粗指甲纹。残损裂，修复后完整。口径较大，大型贮藏器。陕西省咸阳市征集。

陕西医史博物馆藏

Pottery Urn

Han Dynasty

Pottery

Mouth Diameter 66 cm/ Bottom Diameter 28 cm/ Height 95 cm

This pottery urn has a round and thick mouth rim, a round body and a flat bottom. There are short and thick nail patterns on the upper part of its belly. This big wide-mouthed container was cracked, but remains intact after repair. It was collected from Xianyang, Shaanxi Province.

Preserved in Shaanxi Museum of Medical History

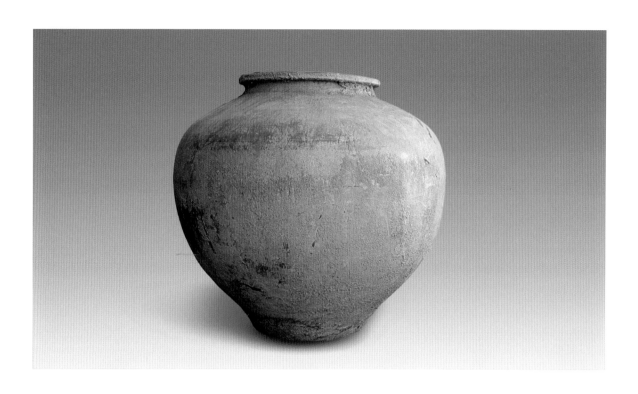

陶瓿

汉

陶质

口径 31 厘米，底径 26.5 厘米，高 54.5 厘米，
重 2590 克

平口沿，圆腹，平底，灰陶，素面。口沿稍残。
盛贮器。陕西省澄城县征集。

陕西医史博物馆藏

Pottery Urn

Han Dynasty

pottery

Mouth Diameter 31 cm/ Bottom Diameter 26.5 cm/
Height 54.5 cm/ Weight 2,590 g

This grey pottery urn, with no decorations, has a
flat mouth rim, a round body and a flat bottom. Its
mouth rim is slightly damaged. The urn was used
as a container and was collected in Chengcheng
County, Shaanxi Province.

Preserved in Shaanxi Museum of Medical History

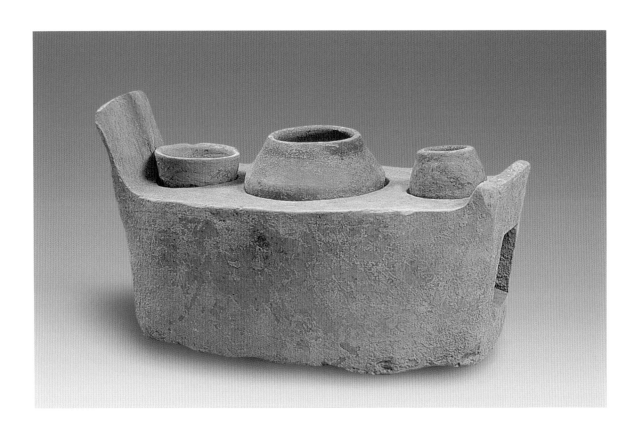

陶灶

汉

陶质

长 37.5 厘米，腰宽 15 厘米，高 8.5 厘米

Pottery Stove

Han Dynasty

Pottery

Length 37.5 cm/ Waist Width 15 cm/ Height 8.5 cm

灶体呈梯形，腹部微鼓，灶面有三个火眼，其上分置锅、釜、甑，灶的一端开有长方形灶门。该灶器形规整，做工精美，又反映了汉代南京地区先民饮食的丰富性。

南京市六合区文物保管所藏

The cross section of the stove is in the shape of a trapezoid. The stove has a slightly swelling belly. On the stove are three burners, on which are placed a pot, a kettle and a rice steamer respectively. On one side of the stove is a rectangular stove opening. The vessel is neat in shape and elegant in workmanship. Besides, it suggests that the people living in Nanjing in the Han Dynasty enjoyed a rich variety of diet. Preserved in Institute of Cultural Relics in Liuhe District, Nanjing City

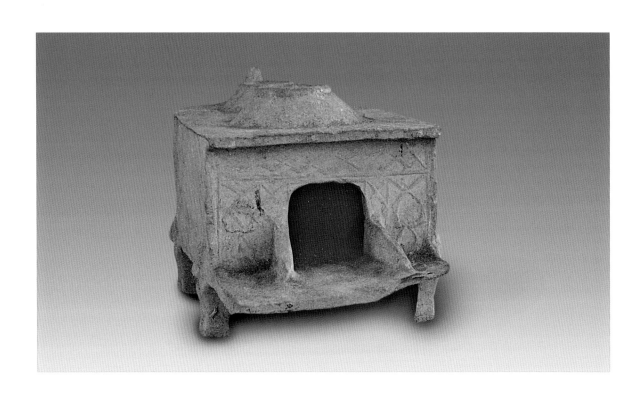

陶灶

汉

陶质

口径 28.5 厘米，宽 15 厘米，通高 12.5 厘米，
重 1900 克

双灶头，带一小锅，一个烟囱，四鼠足。有残。
炊器。陕西省西安市长安区征集。

陕西医史博物馆藏

Pottery Stove

Han Dynasty

Pottery

Mouth Diameter 28.5 cm/ Width 15 cm/ Height
12.5 cm/ Weight 1,900 g

The stove, slightly damaged, has double kitchen
burners, a small pan, a chimney and four rat-shaped
feet. It was used as a cooking vessel, and was
collected in Chang'an District of Xi'an, Shaanxi
Province.

Preserved in Shaanxi Museum of Medical History

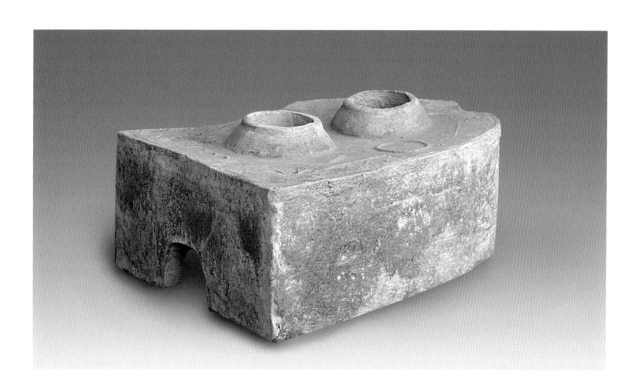

黄釉陶灶

汉

陶质

长 19 厘米，高 8.5 厘米，灶头宽 14.8 厘米，重 1200 克

半椭圆形，两灶头，灶面上有图案。有残。炊器。陕西省澄城县征集。

陕西医史博物馆藏

Yellow-glazed Pottery Stove

Han Dynasty

Pottery

Length 19 cm/ Height 8.5 cm/ Width of The Kitchen Burner 14.8 cm/ Weight 1,200 g

The semi-oval stove has double kitchen burners, with its face decorated with designs. The collection, slightly damaged, was used as a cooking vessel, and was collected in Chengcheng County, Shaanxi Province.

Preserved in Shaanxi Museum of Medical History

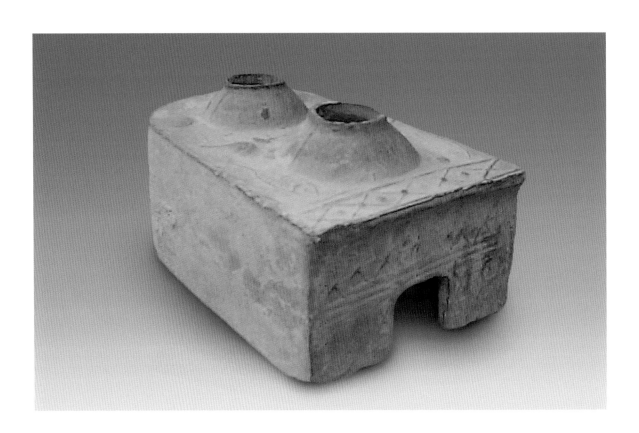

陶灶

汉

陶质

上口径 3.4/3.2 厘米，长 21.2 厘米 ，大头 14.9 厘米 ×11.9 厘米，小头 11.7 厘米 ×11.2 厘米

Pottery Stove

Han Dynasty

Pottery

Upper Mouth Diameter 3.4,3.2 cm/ Length 21.2 cm/ Larger Burner 14.9 cm×11.9 cm/ Smaller Burner 11.7 cm×11.2 cm

该藏由灰陶制成，上部有两灶眼，一端有灶口，工艺一般。长方状，为明器陶灶。保存基本完好。1978 年入藏。

中华医学会 / 上海中医药大学医史博物馆藏

The rectangular vessel was made of grey pottery On its top are two burners, and on one side of the stove is an opening. The stove, with ordinary craftsmanship, was a burial object and has basically been kept in good shape. It was collected in the year 1978.

Preserved in Chinese Medical Association/ Museum of Chinese Medicine, Shanghai University of Traditional Chinese Medicine

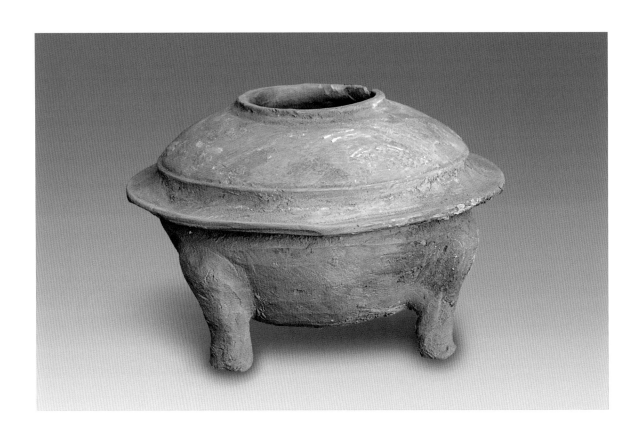

陶鼎

汉

陶质

口径 7 厘米，足高 6.5 厘米，通高 12.3 厘米，重 1000 克

Pottery "Ding" (Tripod)

Han Dynasty

Pottery

Mouth Diameter 7 cm/ Foot Height 6.5 cm/ Height 12.3 cm/ Weight 1,000 g

圆口，腹有一卷沿，圆底，三蹄足，灰陶上饰有彩绘。口沿略残。生活用器。陕北征集。

陕西医史博物馆藏

This "Ding" has a round mouth, a round bottom and three horseshoe-shaped feet. Its belly is surrounded by a circle of rolled edge. With its mouth rim slightly damaged, the grey pottery object is decorated with coloured paintings. The collection served as a household utensil, and was collected in Northern Shaanxi.

Preserved in Shaanxi Museum of Medical History

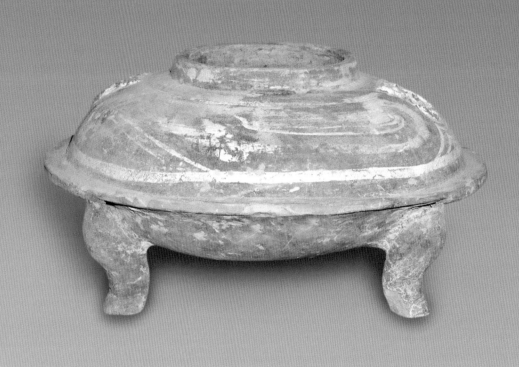

彩绘陶鼎

汉

陶质

口径 8.5 厘米，足高 5 厘米，通高 11 厘米， 重 1050 克

直圆口，圆肩，三蹄足，肩部兽首衔环浮雕双耳，腹中部折沿。完整无损。明器。陕北征集。

陕西医史博物馆藏

Painted Pottery "Ding" (Tripod)

Han Dynasty

Pottery

Mouth Diameter 8.5 cm/ Foot Height 5 cm/ Height 11 cm/ Weight 1,050 g

The pottery "Ding" has a straight round mouth, a rounded shoulder and three horseshoe-shaped feet. On its shoulder is decorated with double handles of relief patterns of animal heads with rings in their mouths. In the middle of its belly is a band raised outer ridge. The well-preserved tripod served as a burial object, and was collected in Northern Shaanxi.

Preserved in Shaanxi Museum of Medical History

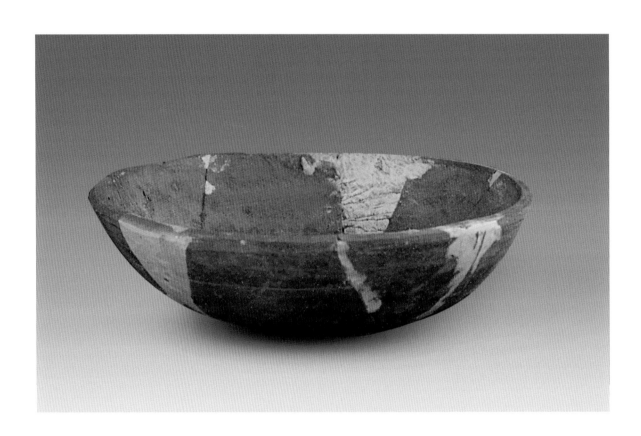

陶鼎盖

汉

陶质

口径 17 厘米，通高 5.5 厘米，重 400 克

Lid of Pottery "Ding" (Tripod)

Han Dynasty

Pottery

Mouth Diameter 17 cm/ Height 5.5 cm/ Weight 400 g

盖为半圆体状，顶有三乳丁，有少量红彩绘。

多处修补。生活用器。陕西省长安区红庆村。

陕西医史博物馆藏

This lid is in the shape of a hemisphere, with three little nails and some red drawings on its top. It was used as a household utensil, and has been repaired in several places. This collection was unearthed from Hongqing Village in Chang'an District, Shaanxi Province.

Preserved in Shaanxi Museum of Medical History

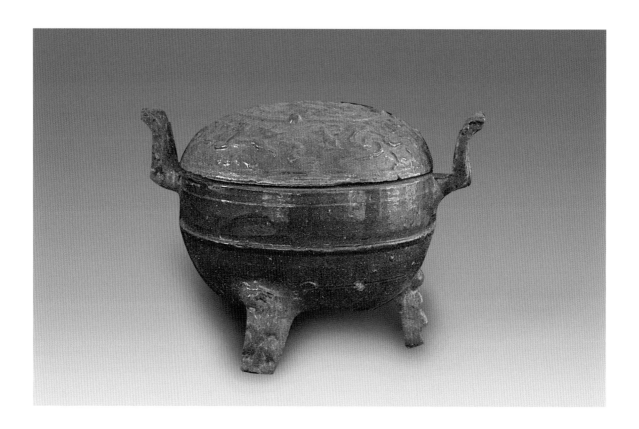

陶簋

汉

釉陶质

口径 15 厘米，通高 18 厘米，足高 7 厘米，重 2150 克

Pottery "Gui" (Food Vessel)

Han Dynasty

Glazed Pottery

Mouth Diameter 15 cm/ Height 18 cm/ Foot Height 7 cm/ Weight 2,150 g

子母口，鼓腹，附耳，三兽足，圆底带盖，
盖有浮雕。完整无损。明器，食器，礼器，
生活器具。陕西省咸阳市窑店胡春芳上交。

陕西医史博物馆藏

This pottery "Gui" has a snap lid with high
reliefs, a globular body, a pair of bail handles,
three beast-shaped feet, and a round bottom.
The well-preserved vessel served as a burial
object, a piece of tableware, a sacrificial vessel,
and a household utensil. It was donated by Hu
Chunfang who lives in Yaodian Sub-district of
Xianyang City, Shaanxi Province.
Preserved in Shaanxi Museum of Medical History

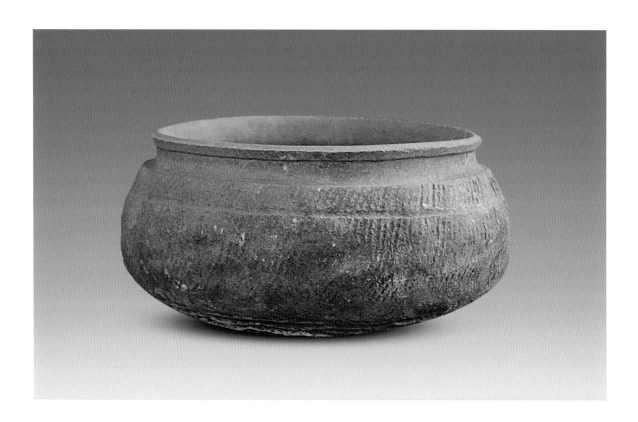

陶釜

汉

陶质

口径 17.5 厘米，底径 11 厘米，通高 9.6 厘米，重 1350 克

Pottery "Fu"(Kettle)

Han Dynasty

Pottery

Mouth Diameter 17.5 cm/ Bottom 11 cm/ Height 9.6 cm/ Weight 1,350 g

侈口，颈腹，周身绳纹，底为粗索纹。完整
无损。生活用器具，炊具。

陕西医史博物馆藏

The mouth of this kettle flares. Its neck, belly
and body are covered with cord patterns, while
its bottom is embellished with thick cable
designs. It remains intact and was used as a
cooking utensil.

Preserved in Shaanxi Museum of Medical History

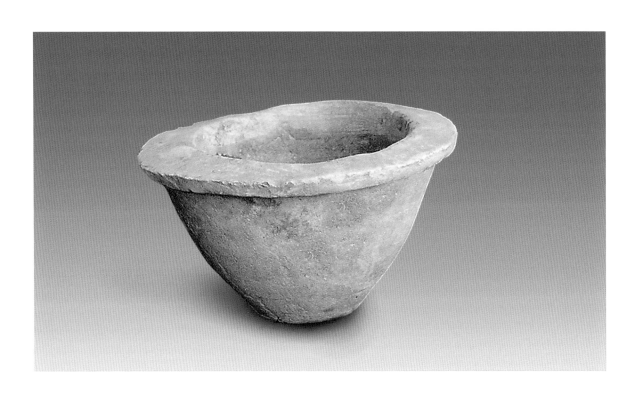

陶甑

汉

陶质

口径 8 厘米，底径 2.5 厘米，高 4.4 厘米，重
100 克

平口沿，斜腹，平底，底有五孔，甑内施有黄釉。
完整无损。炊器。陕西省澄城县征集。

陕西医史博物馆藏

Pottery "Zeng" (Steamer)

Han Dynasty

Pottery

Mouth Diameter 8 cm/ Bottom Diameter 2.5 cm/
Height 4.4 cm/ Weight 100 g

This steamer, a cooking vessel, has a flat mouth
rim, the body tapering to a flat bottom on which are
five holes. The interior of the steamer is covered
with yellow glaze. This cooking vessel is well-
preserved, and was collected from Chengcheng
County, Shaanxi Province.

Preserved in Shaanxi Museum of Medical History

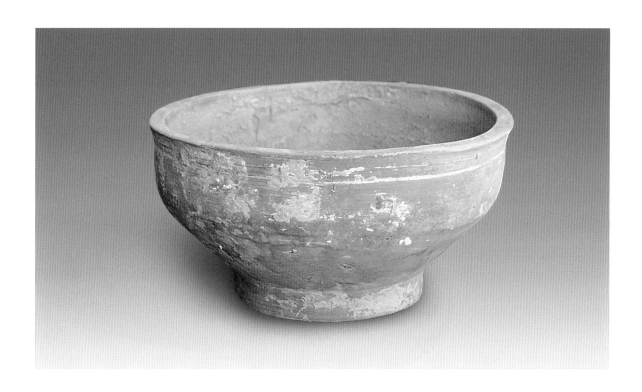

陶甑

汉

陶质

口径 20 厘米，底径 10.5 厘米，高 10 厘米，重
750 克

直口，平口沿，折腹，圈足，甑底有不规则口眼，
灰陶。完整无损。炊器。陕西省澄城县征集。

陕西医史博物馆藏

Pottery "Zeng" (Steamer)

Han Dynasty

Pottery

Mouth Diameter 20 cm/ Base Diameter 10.5 cm/
Height 10 cm/ Weight 750 g

This grey pottery food steamer, a cooking vessel,
has a straight mouth with a flat rim, a tapering
ovoid body and a ring foot. On the bottom of the
steamer are irregular holes. The collection remains
intact, and was collected from Chengcheng County,
Shaanxi Province.

Preserved in Shaanxi Museum of Medical History

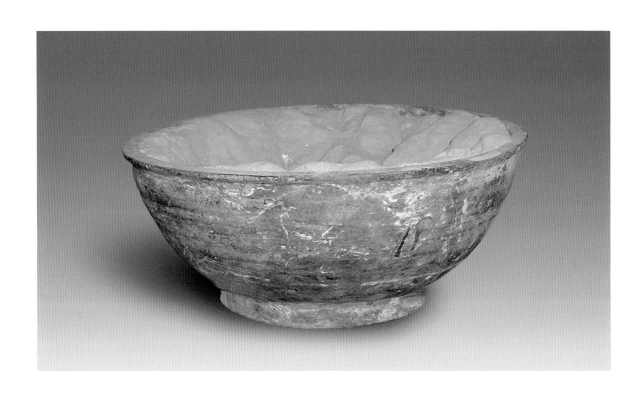

彩绘陶甑

汉

陶质

口径 20.5 厘米，底径 10.9 厘米，高 8 厘米，重
650 克

平口沿，斜腹，圈足，外部有六道彩色弦纹，灰
陶。底残。炊器。陕北征集。

陕西医史博物馆藏

Painted Pottery "Zeng" (Steamer)

Han Dynasty

Pottery

Mouth Diameter 20.5 cm/ Base Diameter 10.9 cm/
Height 8 cm/ Weight 650 g

This grey pottery steamer, has a flat mouth rim, a
tapering ovoid body, and a ring foot. On the exterior
wall are six rings of colourful bowstring patterns.
The cooking vessel has a cracked bottom, and was
collected from northern Shaanxi Province.

Preserved in Shaanxi Museum of Medical History

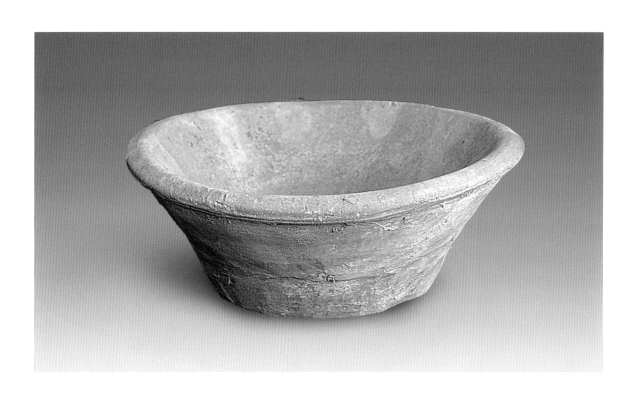

陶碗

汉

陶质

口径 20 厘米，底径 11.6 厘米，高 7 厘米，重
1150 克

敞口，斜腹，平底，灰陶。完整无损。食器。陕
西省澄城县征集。

陕西医史博物馆藏

Pottery Bowl

Han Dynasty

Pottery

Mouth Diameter 20 cm/ Bottom Diameter 11.6 cm/
Height 7 cm/ Weight 1,150 g

This grey pottery bowl, a food container, has a
flared mouth, a body tapering to the flat bottom. It is
preserved well and was collected from Chengcheng
County, Shaanxi Province.

Preserved in Shaanxi Museum of Medical History

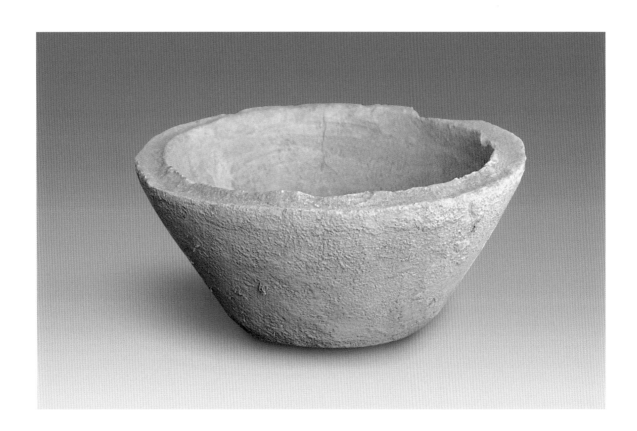

陶碗

汉

陶质

口径 16.5 厘米，底径 8.4 厘米，高 7 厘米，重 700 克

Pottery Bowl

Han Dynasty

Pottery

Mouth Diameter 16.5 cm/ Bottom Diameter 8.4 cm/ Height 7 cm/ Weight 700 g

平口沿，敞口，斜腹，平底，素面，灰陶。
口沿残。食器。陕西省澄城县征集。

陕西医史博物馆藏

Without any decoration, this grey pottery bowl

has a flared mouth, a flat rim that is cracked,

a body tapering to the flat bottom. It served

as a food container and was collected from

Chengcheng County, Shaanxi Province.

Preserved in Shaanxi Museum of Medical History

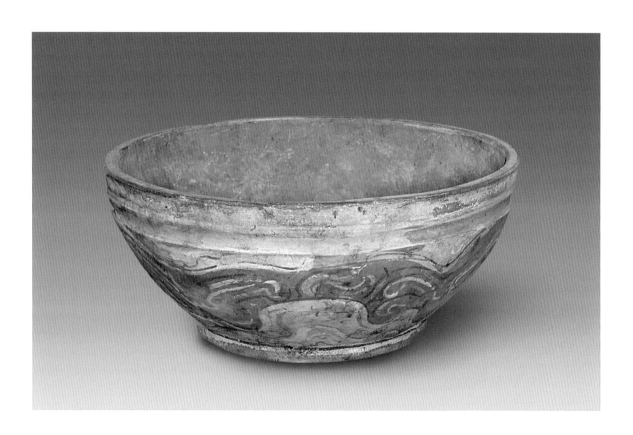

彩绘陶碗

汉

陶质

口径 18 厘米，底径 10.3 厘米，高 7.5 厘米，重 500 克

Painted Pottery Bowl

Han Dynasty

Pottery

Mouth Diameter 18 cm/ Bottom Diameter 10.3 cm/ Height 7.5 cm/ Weight 500 g

直口，斜腹，浅圈足，碗沿下 1 厘米处，有一道凹纹，通身彩绘，灰陶。完整无损。生活器具。陕北征集。

陕西医史博物馆藏

This grey pottery bowl, a piece of household ware, has a straight mouth, a body tapering to a shallow ring foot. One centimeter below the mouth rim is found a concave line. The whole body is decorated with coloured drawings. It is preserved well and was collected from northern Shaanxi Province.

Preserved in Shaanxi Museum of Medical History

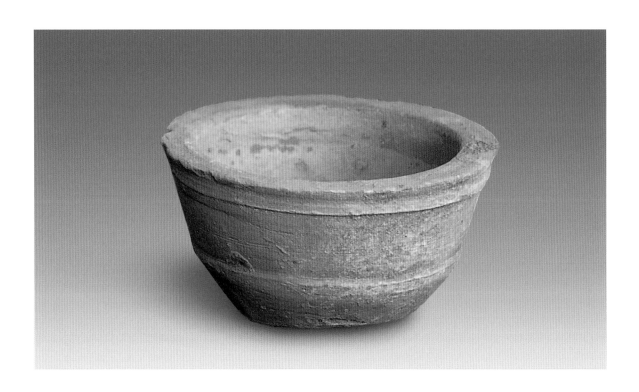

陶盆

汉

红陶质

口径 10 厘米，底径 5.5 厘米，高 4.8 厘米，重 200 克

平口沿，直斜腹，平底，红陶，素面。完整无损。生活器具。陕西省澄城县征集。

陕西医史博物馆藏

Pottery Pot

Han Dynasty

Red Pottery

Mouth Diameter 10 cm/ Bottom Diameter 5.5 cm/ Height 4.8 cm/ Weight 200 g

This pot, a piece of household ware with no decoration, has a flat mouth rim, a straight body tapering the flat bottom. It is preserved well and was collected from Chengcheng County, Shaanxi Province.

Preserved in Shaanxi Museum of Medical History

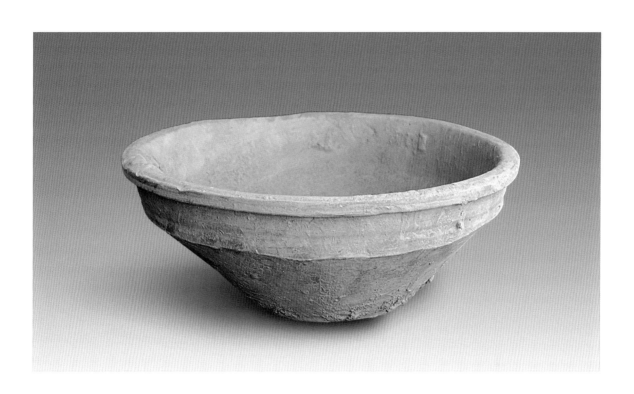

陶盆

汉

陶质

口径 27.5 厘米，底径 12.5 厘米，高 10.6 厘米，重 1500 克

敞口，直肩，斜腹，平底，灰陶。口沿残。盛贮器。陕西省澄城县征集。

陕西医史博物馆藏

Pottery Pot

Han Dynasty

Pottery

Mouth Diameter 27.5 cm/ Bottom Diameter 12.5 cm/ Height 10.6 cm/ Weight 1,500 g

This grey pottery pot for storage has a flared mouth with a cracked rim, a straight shoulder, and a body tapering to a flat bottom. The object was collected from Chengcheng County, Shaanxi Province.

Preserved in Shaanxi Museum of Medical History

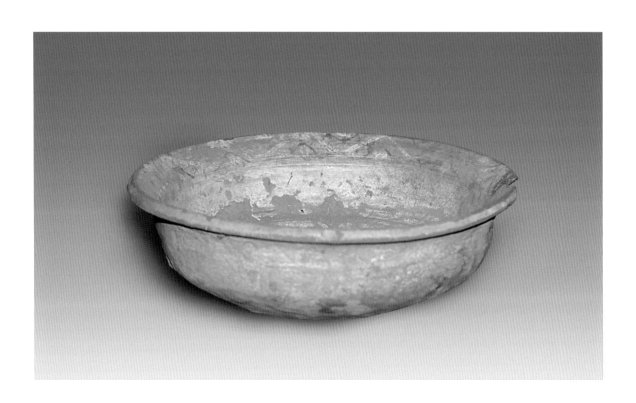

彩绘陶盆

汉

陶质

口径 19.4 厘米，底径 8.5 厘米，高 6 厘米，重
450 克

敞口，折腹，平底，盆内有彩绘，灰陶。口沿残。
生活器具。陕北征集。

陕西医史博物馆藏

Painted Pottery Basin

Han Dynasty

Grey Pottery

Mouth Diameter 19.4 cm/ Bottom Diameter 8.5 cm/
Height 6 cm/ Weight 450 g

This grey pottery basin, a piece of household ware,
has a flared mouth with a cracked rim, a tapering
ovoid body, and a flat bottom. The interior of
the basin is decorated with coloured drawings.
The object was collected from northern Shaanxi
Province.

Preserved in Shaanxi Museum of Medical History

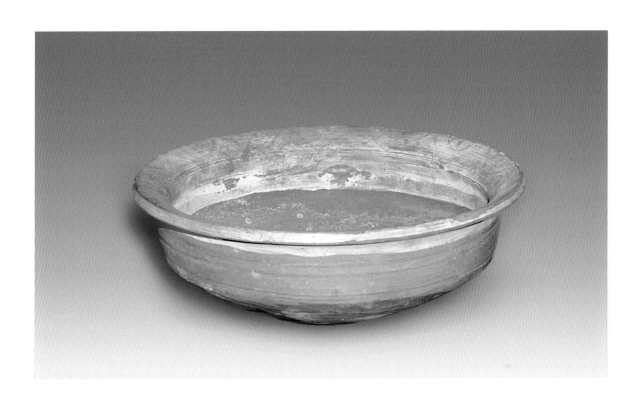

彩绘陶盆

汉

陶质

口径 16.5 厘米，底径 7 厘米，高 5.2 厘米，重
30 克

敞口，折腹，平底，灰陶，口沿和盆内有彩绘。
完整无损。生活器具。陕北征集。

陕西医史博物馆藏

Painted Pottery Basin

Han Dynasty

Pottery

Mouth Diameter 16.5 cm/ Bottom Diameter 7 cm/
Height 5.2 cm/ Weight 30 g

This grey pottery pot, a piece of household ware,
has a flared mouth, a tapering ovoid body, and a
flat bottom. The mouth rim and the interior wall
are decorated with coloured drawings. The pot,
still in good condition, was collected from northern
Shaanxi Province.

Preserved in Shaanxi Museum of Medical History

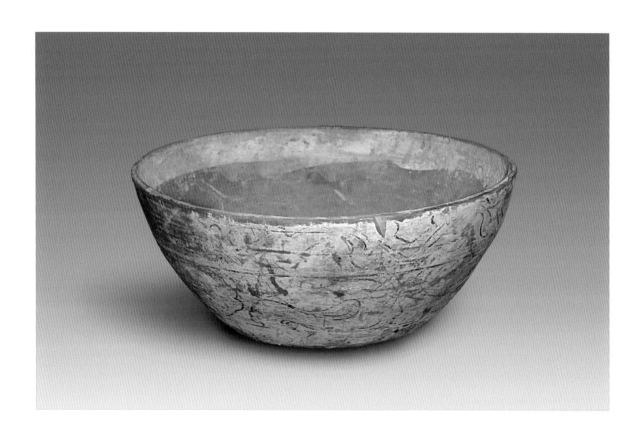

彩绘陶盆

汉

陶质

口径 20 厘米，底径 11 厘米，高 7.6 厘米，重 700 克

Painted Pottery Basin

Han Dynasty

Pottery

Mouth Diameter 20 cm/ Bottom Diameter 11 cm/ Height 7.6 cm/ Weight 700 g

敞口，直斜腹，平底，通身彩绘，灰陶。完
整无损。生活器具。陕北征集。

陕西医史博物馆藏

This grey pottery basin, a piece of household
ware, has a flared mouth, a straight body
tapering to a flat bottom. Its whole body is
decorated with coloured drawings. The basin,
which is kept intact, was collected from
northern Shaanxi Province.

Preserved in Shaanxi Museum of Medical History

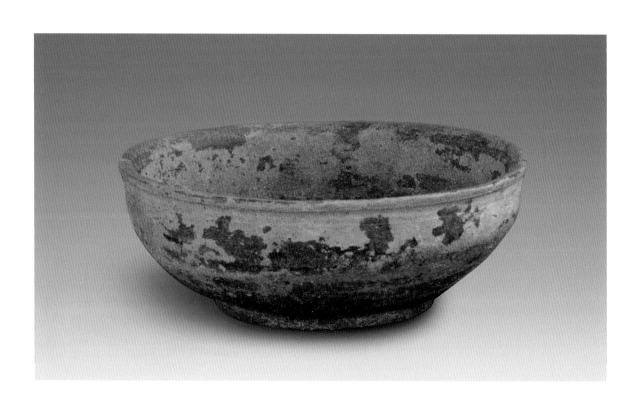

陶钵

汉

陶质

口径 19.5 厘米，通高 7.5 厘米，底径 10.2 厘米，
重 500 克

敞口，垂腹，假圈足。完整无损。食具，生活用
具。陕西省西安市长安区康申利上交征集。

陕西医史博物馆藏

Pottery Bowl

Han Dynasty

Pottery

Mouth Diameter 19.5 cm/ Height 7.5 cm/ Bottom
Diameter 10.2 cm/ Weight 500 g

This bowl, a food container, has a flared mouth and
a tapering ovoid body, with a fake ring foot as its
bottom. The object remains intact, and was donated
by Kang Shenli from Chang'an District, Xi'an city,
Shaanxi Province.

Preserved in Shaanxi Museum of Medical History

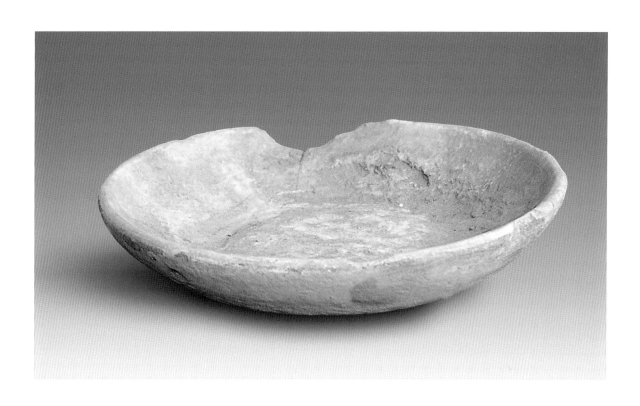

陶盘

汉

陶质

口径 16 厘米，底径 11 厘米，高 2.5 厘米，重
2500 克

敞口，平底，灰陶，素面。口沿残。生活器具。
陕西省澄城县征集。

陕西医史博物馆藏

Pottery Plate

Han Dynasty

Pottery

Mouth Diameter 16 cm/ Bottom Diameter 11 cm/
Height 2.5 cm/ Weight 2,500 g

This grey pottery plate, a piece of household
ware with no decoration, has a flared mouth with
a cracked rim and a flat bottom. The object was
collected from Chengcheng County, Shaanxi
Province.

Preserved in Shaanxi Museum of Medical History

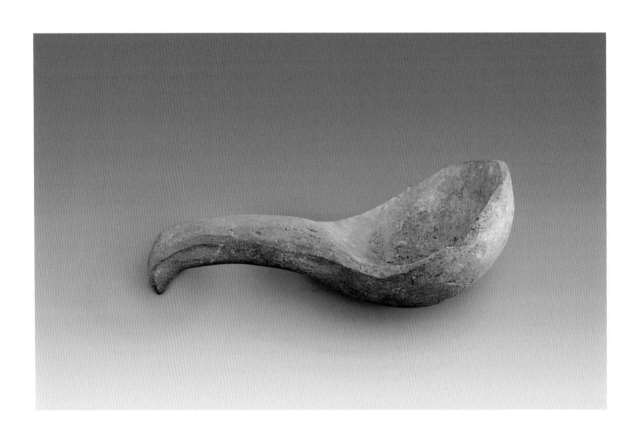

陶勺

汉

陶质

口径 7 厘米，通高 3 厘米，重 100 克

勺状，圆底，把为勾形。完整无损。生活用器具，

食器。

陕西医史博物馆藏

Pottery Spoon

Han Dynasty

Pottery

Mouth Diameter 7 cm/ Height 3 cm/ Weight 100 g

This spoon, a piece of tableware, has a round
bottom and a hook-shaped handle. The object
remains intact.

Preserved in Shaanxi Museum of Medical History

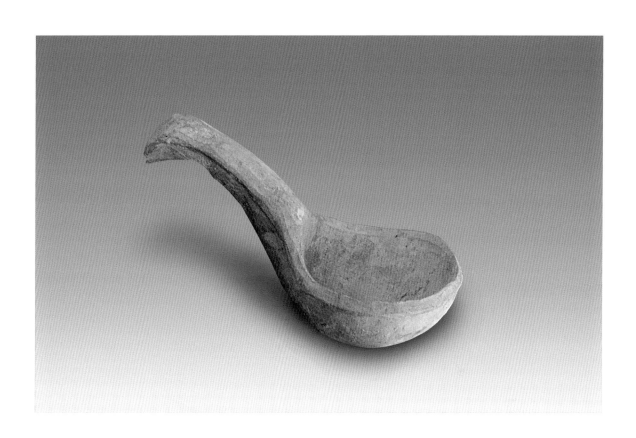

陶勺

汉

陶质

口径 7 厘米，通高 3 厘米，重 100 克

勺状，圆底，把为钩形。完整无损。生活用器具，

食器。陕西省长安区征集。

陕西医史博物馆藏

Pottery Spoon

Han Dynasty

Pottery

Mouth Diameter 7 cm/ Height 3 cm/ Weight 100 g

This spoon, a piece of tableware, has a round bottom and a hook-shaped handle. It has been preserved well and was collected from Chang'an District, Shaanxi Province.

Preserved in Shaanxi Museum of Medical History

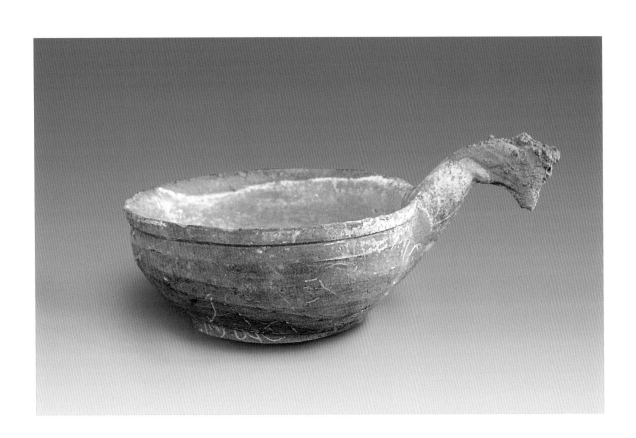

陶勺

汉

陶质

口径 17 厘米，底径 10 厘米，通高 7.5 厘米，重 600 克

侈口，圆腹，假圈足，口沿处有一把为鸟头。完整无损。生活用器具，食器。

陕西医史博物馆藏

Pottery Spoon

Han Dynasty

Pottery

Mouth Diameter 17 cm/ Bottom Diameter 10 cm/ Height 7.5 cm/ Weight 600 g

This spoon, a piece of tableware, has a flared mouth, a rounded body and a fake ring foot. with a bird-head-shaped handle attached to its mouth rim. The object remains intact.

Preserved in Shaanxi Museum of Medical History

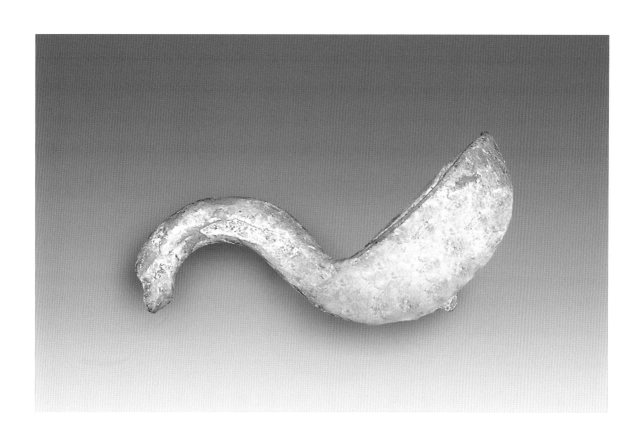

陶勺

汉

白陶质

口径 6 厘米，通高 7.2 厘米，重 50 克

勺状，勺把呈弯曲形状。完整无损。食器，炊器。

陕西省西安市征集。

陕西医史博物馆藏

Pottery Spoon

Han Dynasty

White Pottery

Mouth Diameter 6 cm/ Height 7.2 cm/ Weight 50 g

The spoon has a long curved handle,and remains intact. It is a piece of tableware as well as a cooking vessel. The object was collected from Xi'an city, Shaanxi province.

Preserved in Shaanxi Museum of Medical History

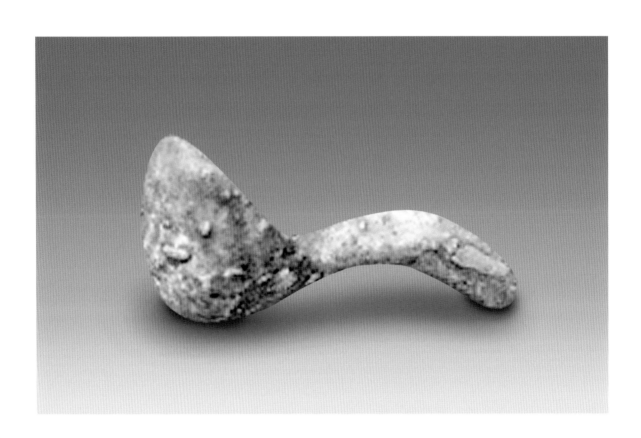

陶勺

汉

陶质

最长 6.7 厘米，最宽 2.8 厘米

长柄。勺状，勺把呈弯曲形状。完整无损。食器，
炊器。

广东中医药博物馆藏

Pottery Spoon

Han Dynasty

Pottery

Maximum Length 6.7 cm/ Maximum Width 2.8 cm

The spoon has a long curved handle. The well-preserved spoon served as a piece of tableware as well as a cooking vessel.

Preserved in Guangdong Chinese Medicine Museum

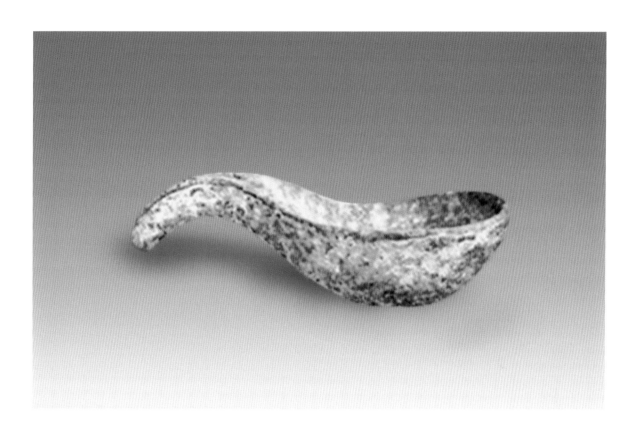

陶勺

汉

陶质

最长 14 厘米，最宽 5.5 厘米

盛物用。勺状。勺把呈弯曲状。食器，炊器。

广东中医药博物馆藏

Pottery Spoon

Han Dynasty

Pottery

Maximum Length 14 cm/ Maximum Width 5.5 cm

The spoon has a curved handle. It is a piece of tableware used to serve food as well as a cooking vessel.

Preserved in Guangdong Chinese Medicine Museum

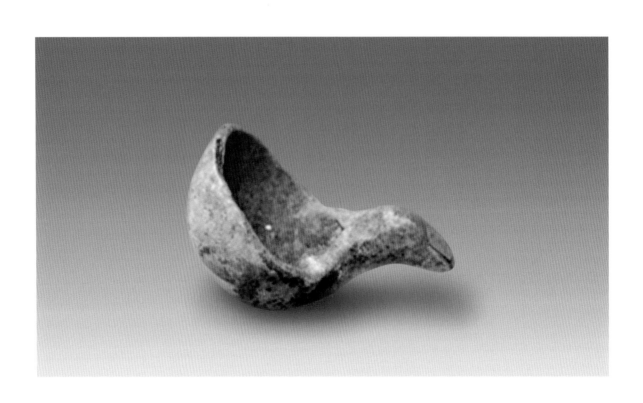

陶勺

汉

陶质

最长 7.5 厘米，最宽 4.8 厘米

盛物用。勺状。食器，炊器。

广东中医药博物馆藏

Pottery Spoon

Han Dynasty

Pottery

Maximum Length 7.5 cm/ Maximum Width 5.5 cm

This spoon was used to serve food.It is a piece of tableware as well as a cooking vessel.

Preserved in Guangdong Chinese Medicine Museum

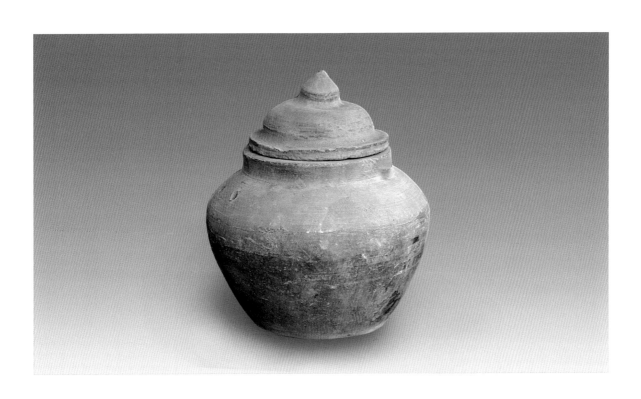

陶温器

汉

陶质

口径 10 厘米，底径 9.3 厘米，高 16.8 厘米，重 1000 克

子母口，溜肩，斜腹，平底，肩部有两个注水孔，腹壁双层，灰陶，素面，带一盖。完整无损。温器。陕西省白水县征集。

陕西医史博物馆藏

Pottery Warming Pot

Han Dynasty

Grey Pottery

Mouth Diameter 10 cm/ Bottom Diameter 9.3 cm/ Height 16.8 cm/ Weight 1,000 g

This grey warming pot, without any decoration, has a snap lid, a sloping shoulder and a tapering ovoid body with flat bottom. On its shoulder are two holes for water injection. The wall of its belly is double-layered. It remains intact, and was collected from Baishui County, Shaanxi Province.

Preserved in Shaanxi Museum of Medical History

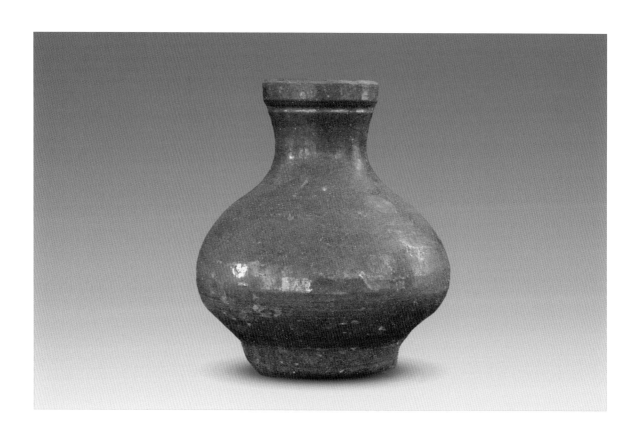

陶钟

汉

黄釉陶质

口径 6.8 厘米，底径 9 厘米，通高 16.5 厘米，重 900 克

Pottery Pot

Han Dynasty

Yellow-glazed Pottery

Mouth Diameter 6.8 cm/ Bottom Diameter 9 cm/ Height 16.5 cm/ Weight 900 g

直口，垂腹，平底。完整无损。盛贮器。陕
西省西安市长安区征集。

陕西医史博物馆藏

This pot for storage has a straight mouth,
a globular body tapering to a flat bottom.
It remains intact and was collected from
the Chang'an District, Xi'an City, Shaanxi
Province.

Preserved in Shaanxi Museum of Medical History

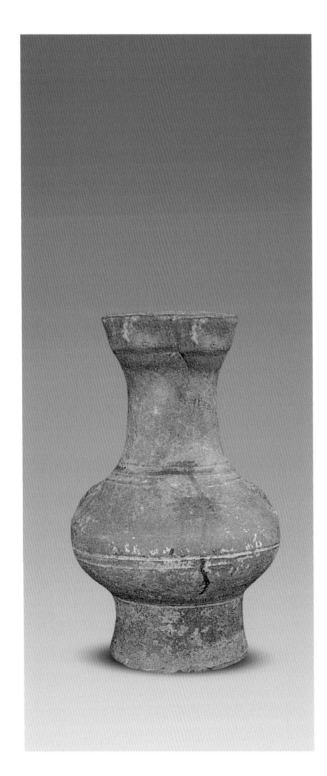

陶钟

汉

绿釉陶质

口径 14 厘米，底径 14.6 厘米，通高 33.5 厘米，
重 2400 克

Pottery Pot

Han Dynasty

Green-glazed Pottery

Mouth Diameter 14 cm/ Base Diameter 14.6 cm/

Height 33.5 cm/ Weight 2,400 g

盘口，长颈，鼓腹，平底，肩部有兽首衔环耳，绿釉。完整无损。容器，礼器。陕西省咸阳市秦都区征集。

陕西医史博物馆藏

This pot has a straight mouth, a long neck, a globular body and a flat base.On the shoulder are moulded beast-head handles with rings in the mouths. The pot served as a container as well as a ritual object. It remains intact, and was collected from the Qindu District, Xianyang City, Shaanxi Province.

Preserved in Shaanxi Museum of Medical History

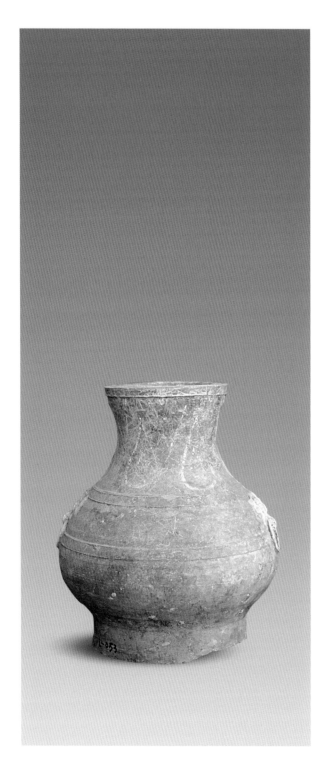

陶钟

汉

陶质

口径 13 厘米，底径 17 厘米，高 27 厘米，重 2300 克

Pottery Pot

Han Dynasty

Pottery

Mouth Diameter 13 cm/ Bottom Diameter 17 cm/ Height 27 cm/ Weight 2,300 g

直口，溜肩，圆腹，假圈足，肩部有兽首衔
环双耳、肩、腹部有两道棱，钟面施有彩绘，
灰陶。底残。生活器具。陕北征集。

陕西医史博物馆藏

This grey pottery pot, a piece of household
ware, has a straight mouth, a sloping shoulder,
a globular body, with a fake ring foot as its
bottom. On the shoulder are moulded beast-head
handles with rings in the mouths. Two ridge
lines are carved on both its shoulder and belly.
Its exterior is decorated with coloured drawings.
The bottom is cracked. The pot was collected
from northern Shaanxi Province.

Preserved in Shaanxi Museum of Medical History

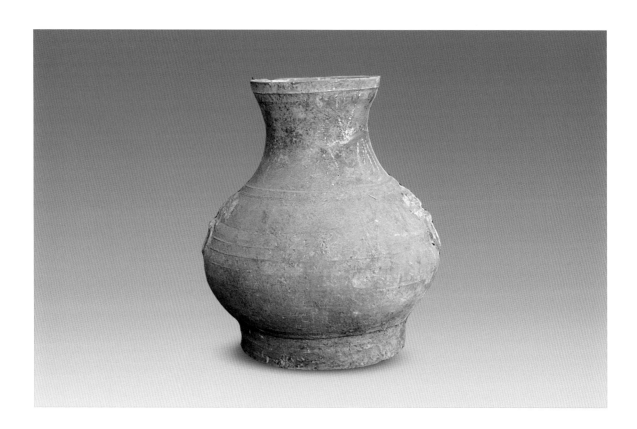

陶钟

汉

陶质

口径 13 厘米，底径 17 厘米，高 27 厘米，重 100 克

Pottery Pot

Han Dynasty

Pottery

Mouth Diameter 13 cm/ Bottom Diameter 17 cm/ Height 27 cm/ Weight 100 g

直口，溜肩，圆腹，假圈足，肩部有兽首衔

环双耳，肩、腹部有二道棱，钟面施有彩绘，

灰陶。口沿略残。生活器具。陕北征集。

陕西医史博物馆藏

This grey pottery pot, a piece of household ware, has a straight mouth, a sloping shoulder, a rounded body, with a fake ring foot as its bottom. On the shoulder are moulded beast-head handles with rings in the mouths. Two ridge lines are carved on both its shoulder and belly. Its exterior is decorated with coloured drawings. Its mouth rim is slightly damaged. The pot was collected from northern Shaanxi Province. Preserved in Shaanxi Museum of Medical History

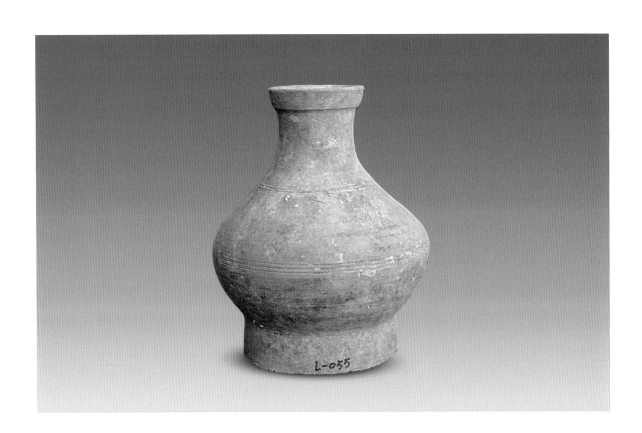

陶钟

汉

陶质

口径 8.5 厘米，底径 14.6 厘米，高 24.1 厘米，重 1550 克

Pottery Pot

Han Dynasty

Pottery

Mouth Diameter 8.5 cm/ Bottom Diameter 14.6 cm/ Height 24.1 cm/ Weight 1,550 g

直口，长颈，溜肩，圆腹，平底，颈、腹部有弦纹，钟面施有彩绘，灰陶。完整无损。生活器具。陕北征集。

陕西医史博物馆藏

The grey pottery pot, a piece of household ware, has a straight mouth, a long neck, a sloping shoulder, a rounded belly and a flat bottom. There are bowstring patterns on its neck and belly. Its exterior is decorated with coloured paintings. The pot remains intact, and was collected from northern Shaanxi Province.

Preserved in Shaanxi Museum of Medical History

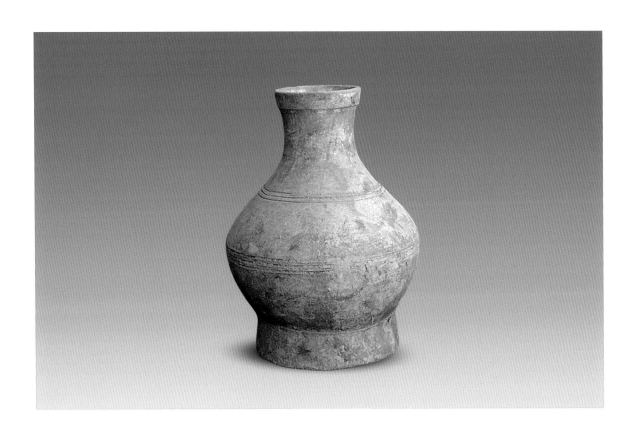

陶钟

汉

陶质

口径 8.5 厘米，底径 14.6 厘米，高 23.1 厘米，重 1800 克

Pottery Pot

Han Dynasty

Pottery

Mouth Diameter 8.5 cm/ Bottom Diameter 14.6 cm/ Height 23.1 cm/ Weight 1,800 g

直口，长颈，溜肩，圆腹，平底，颈、腹部有弦纹，钟面施有彩绘，灰陶。完整无损。生活器具。陕北征集。

陕西医史博物馆藏

This grey pottery pot, a piece of household ware, has a straight mouth, a long neck, a sloping shoulder, a rounded belly and a flat bottom. There are bowstring patterns on its neck and belly. Its exterior surface is decorated with coloured paintings. The pot is kept in good condition, and was collected from northern Shaanxi Province.

Preserved in Shaanxi Museum of Medical History

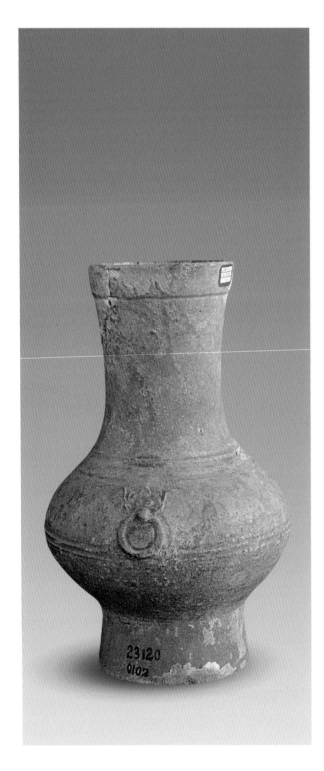

绿釉陶钟

汉

陶质

口径为 15.5 厘米，底径 17 厘米，通高 40 厘米，
重 4600 克

Green-glazed Pottery Pot

Han Dynasty

Pottery

Mouth Diameter 15.5cm/ Bottom Diameter 17cm/

Height 40 cm/ Weight 4,600 g

直口，长颈，鼓腹，平底，肩上有三道弦纹
和兽首衔环耳。口颈有修补。盛酒器，盛水器。
陕西历史博物馆调拨。

陕西医史博物馆藏

The pottery pot has a straight mouth, a long
neck, a globular body, and a flat bottom. Its
shoulder is decorated with three rings of
bowstring patterns and are moulded beast-head
handles with rings in the mouths. The mouth
and neck have been repaired. This collection
served as wine vessel as well as water container.
It was allocated from Shaanxi History Museum.
Preserved in Shaanxi Museum of Medical History

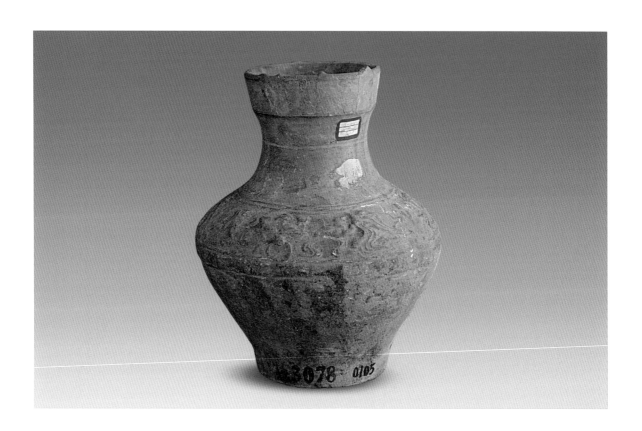

绿釉陶钟

汉

陶质

口径 14 厘米，底径 14 厘米，通高 30 厘米，重 3200 克

Green-glazed Pottery Pot

Han Dynasty

Pottery

Mouth Diameter 14 cm/ Bottom Diameter 14 cm/ Height 30 cm/ Weight 3,200 g

直口，折肩，平底，肩部有动物浮雕图案，
兽首衔环耳。底部有一破洞。盛酒器，盛水器。
陕西历史博物馆调拨。

陕西医史博物馆藏

The pot has a straight mouth, a sloping
shoulder, and a flat bottom with a broken hole.
Its shoulder is decorated with animal patterns
in relief, and are moulded animal-head handles
with rings in the mouths. It was used as a wine
vessel as well as a water container. and was
allocated from Shaanxi History Museum.
Preserved in Shaanxi Museum of Medical History

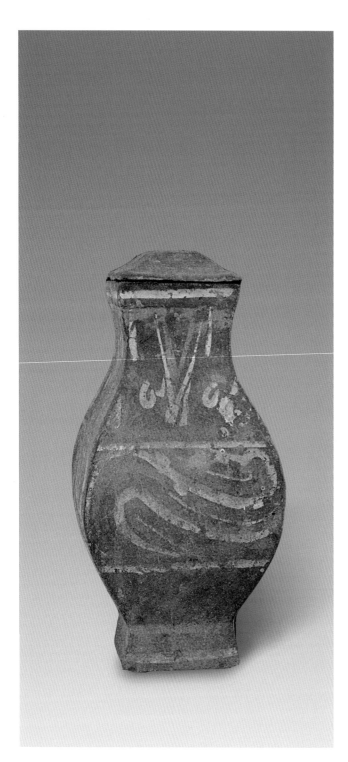

陶钫

汉

陶质

口径10厘米，底径9.5厘米，通高33厘米，
重1650克

Pottery "Fang" (Wine Vessel)

Han Dynasty

Pottery

Mouth Diameter 10 cm/ Base Diameter 9.5 cm/

Height 33 cm/ Weight 1,650 g

子母口，带盖，方形，鼓腹，通体黄白彩绘，
腹部有双耳、浮雕。腹底有修补。酒器。

陕西医史博物馆藏

This wine vessel is cuboid in shape with a snap
lid and a rounded belly. The whole body is
decorated with yellow and white paintings, with
two handles and motifs in relief on the belly. Its
bottom has been repaired.

Preserved in Shaanxi Museum of Medical History

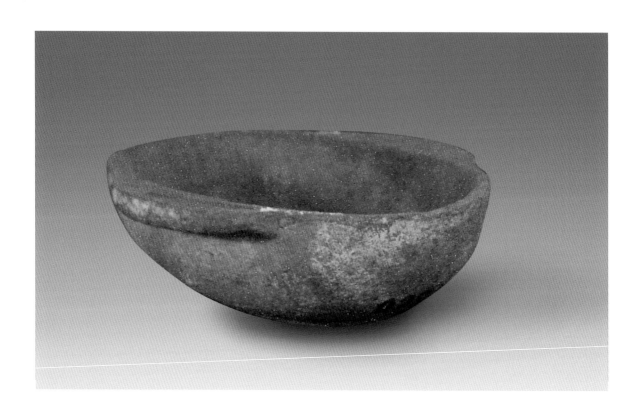

陶耳杯

汉

陶质

口径 10 厘米，宽 8 厘米，通高 3 厘米，重 100 克

椭圆形状，双平耳，平底，无纹饰。完整无损。

酒器。陕西省西安市长安区征集。

陕西医史博物馆藏

Pottery Cup with Handles

Han Dynasty

Pottery

Mouth Diameter 10 cm/ Width 8 cm/ Height 3 cm/
Weight 100 g

This cup is oval in shape. It has a pair of flat
handles and a flat bottom，with no decoration.
Served as a wine vessel, it remains intact. The cup
was collected from Chang'an District, Xi'an City,
Shaanxi Province.

Preserved in Shaanxi Museum of Medical History

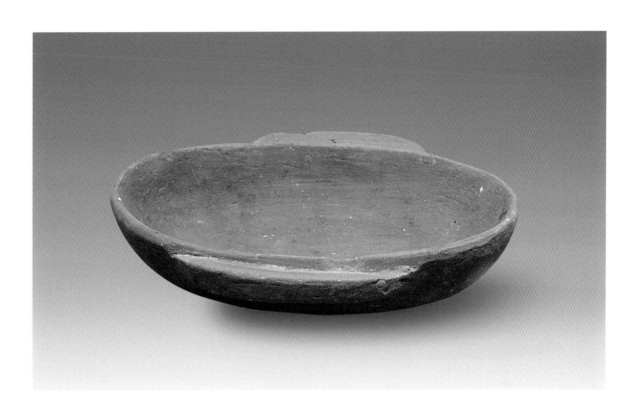

耳杯

汉

陶质

长 18.5 厘米，宽 8 厘米

由红陶制作，是饮酒用具。由成都市考古队调拨。

成都中医药大学中医药传统文化博物馆藏

Handled Cup

Han Dynasty

Pottery

Length 18.5 cm/ Width 8 cm

This red pottery cup was used as a wine vessel. It was allocated from Archaeological Team of Chengdu City.

Preserved in Museum of Traditional Chinese Medicine Culture, Chengdu University of Traditional Chinese Medicine

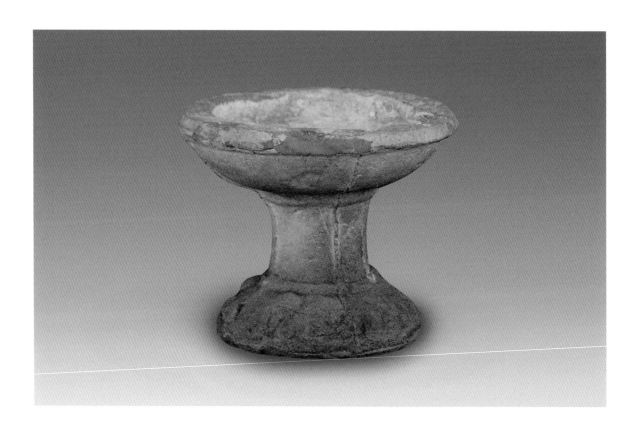

陶豆

汉

陶质

口径 11 厘米，底径 8.5 厘米，通高 9 厘米，重 550 克

Pottery "Dou" (Stemmed Bowl)

Han Dynasty

Pottery

Mouth Diameter 11 cm/ Bottom Diameter 8.5 cm/ Height 9 cm/ Weight 550 g

平沿厚钝，柄粗短，平底。完整无损。食器。

陕西省西安市长安区征集。

陕西医史博物馆藏

The "Dou" has a flat thick mouth rim, a short thick handle and a flat bottom. The bowl served as a food container, and remains intact. It was collected from Chang'an District, Xi'an City, Shaanxi Province.

Preserved in Shaanxi Museum of Medical History

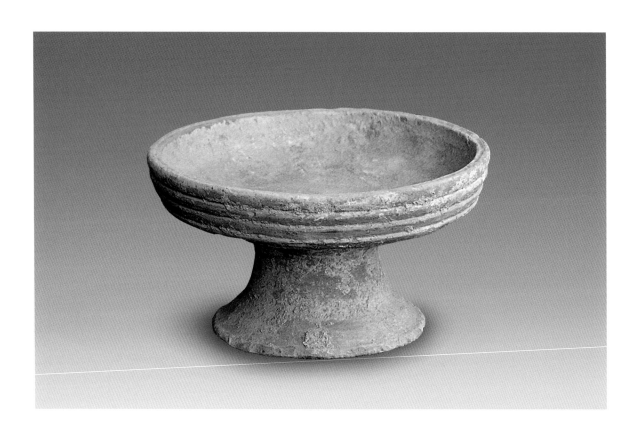

陶豆

汉

陶质

口径 14 厘米，底径 9 厘米，高 7.4 厘米，重 350 克

Pottery "Dou" (Stemmed Bowl)

Han Dynasty

Pottery

Mouth Diameter 14 cm/ Bottom Diameter 9 cm/ Height 7.4 cm/ Weight 350 g

盘口，倒喇叭座，口外沿有三道弦纹，灰陶。
底座略残。生活器具。陕西省澄城县征集。

陕西医史博物馆藏

The "Dou" has a dish-shaped mouth and an
inverted trumpet-shaped bottom, with three
rings of string patterns around the exterior
mouth rim. This grey pottery piece, used as
a daily living utensil, is slightly broken on its
base. It was collected from Chengcheng County,
Shaanxi Province.

Preserved in Shaanxi Museum of Medical History

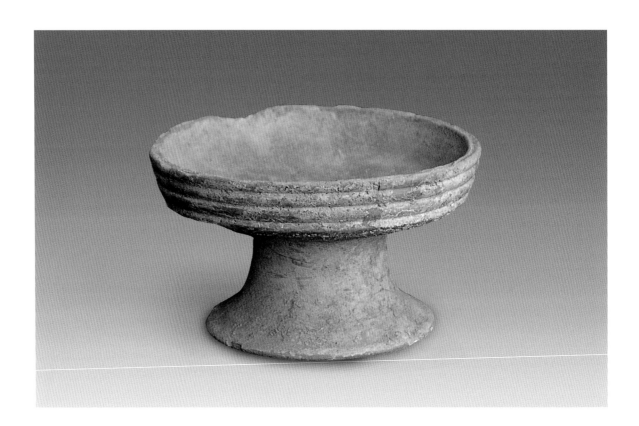

陶豆

汉

陶质

口径 14 厘米，底径 9.8 厘米，高 7.8 厘米，重 400 克

Pottery "Dou" (Stemmed Bowl)

Han Dynasty

Pottery

Mouth Diameter 14 cm/ Bottom Diameter 9.8 cm/ Height 7.8 cm/ Weight 400 g

盘口，倒喇叭口，口沿外有三道弦纹，灰陶。

口沿略残。生活器具。陕西省澄城县征集。

　　　　　　　　　　　陕西医史博物馆藏

The "Dou" has a dish-shaped mouth and an
inverted trumpet-shaped bottom, with three
rings of string patterns around the exterior
mouth rim. This grey pottery piece, used as a
daily living utensil, is slightly broken on its
mouth rim. It was collected from Chengcheng
County, Shaanxi Province.

Preserved in Shaanxi Museum of Medical History

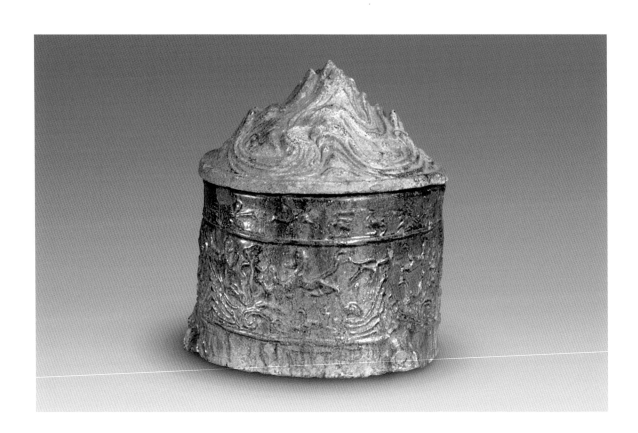

绿釉禽兽纹陶奁

汉

陶质

高 24.5 厘米，口径 22 厘米

Green Glazed "Lian" (Dressing Case) with Beast Patterns

Han Dynasty

Pottery

Height 24.5 cm/ Mouth Diameter 22 cm

直腹，平底，三足，上有盖，盖饰博山状。通体施绿釉，釉色光亮。腹外壁饰凸弦纹二周，将腹部分成两个装饰带。上饰动物纹环器口一周，下为两组相同图案，有山、兽、鸟等。两组图案由竖弦纹相隔。

山西博物院藏

Covered with bright green glaze, the "Lian" (dressing case) has a straight body, a flat bottom, three feet and a Boshan-style lid. Around the exterior wall of the belly are two tiers of convex string patterns which divide the belly into two bands of decoration. The upper part close to the mouth is decorated with a circle of beast patterns, while the lower part with two sets of the same motifs, including mountains, beasts, birds and the like, separated by vertical string patterns.

Preserved in Shaanxi Museum

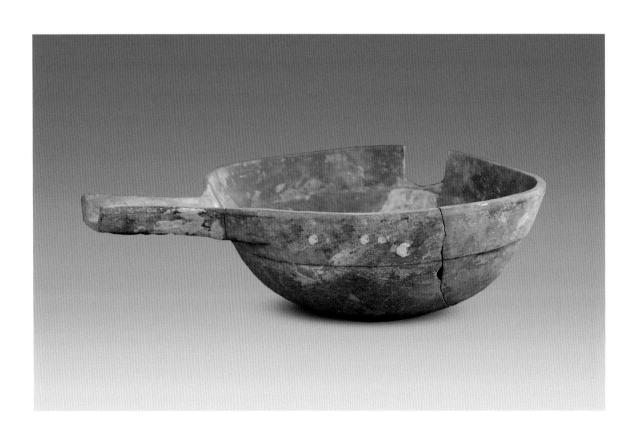

陶匜

汉

陶质

口径 25 厘米，通高 10 厘米，底径 13 厘米，重 1000 克

Pottery "Yi" (Gourd-shaped Ladle)

Han Dynasty

Pottery

Mouth Diameter 25 cm/ Height 10 cm/ Bottom Diameter 13 cm/ Weight 1,000 g

侈口，方体平底，开流，流对面处腹有一兽
首衔环浮雕。有残，有修补。生活用器具。
陕西省咸阳市博物馆调拨。

陕西医史博物馆藏

The ladle has a flaring mouth, a square body, a
flat bottom, and a spout. To the opposite of the
spout is moulded a relief of a beast head with
a ring in the mouth. This "Yi", a household
utensil for daily use, is damaged and has been
restored. It was allocated from Xianyang
Museum, Shaanxi Province.

Preserved in Shaanxi Museum of Medical History

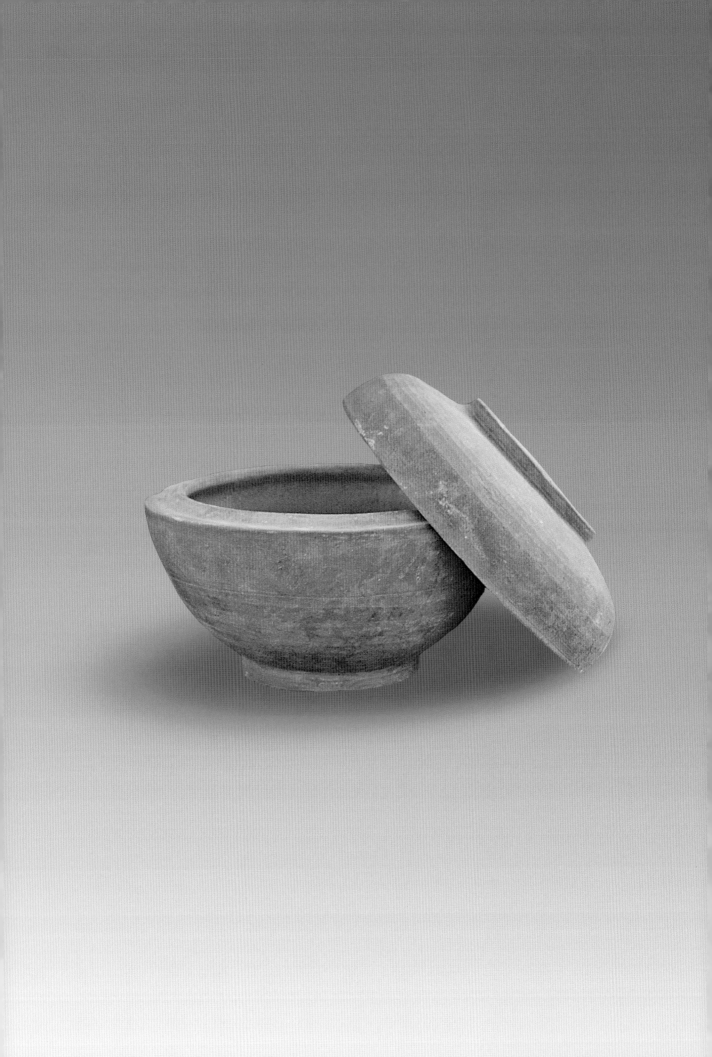

陶盒

汉

陶质

口径 19 厘米，底径 9.5 厘米，通高 15 厘米，重 1200 克

子母口，圆腹，圈足，带一盒盖。完整无损。生活用器具，盛贮器。陕西省长安区红庆村征集。

陕西医史博物馆藏

Pottery Box

Han Dynasty

Pottery

Mouth Diameter 19 cm/ Bottom Diameter 9.5 cm/ Height 15 cm/ Weight 1,200 g

This box has a snap lid, a rounded belly, tapering to a ring foot. This box, a household utensil for daily use, remains intact. It was collected from Hongqing Village, Chang'an District, Shaanxi Province.

Preserved in Shaanxi Museum of Medical History

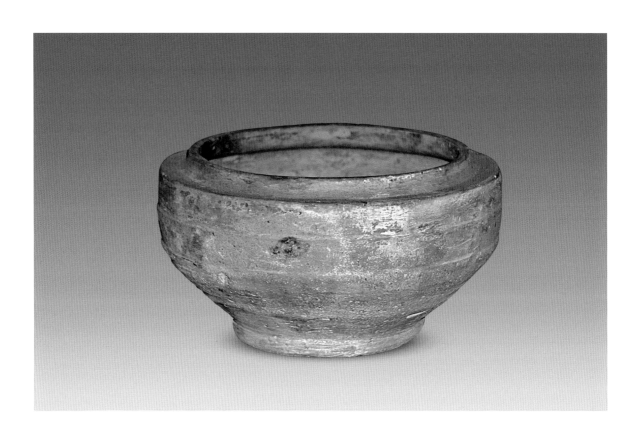

陶盒

汉

陶质

口径 17.8 厘米，底径 10 厘米，通高 10 厘米，重 750 克

Pottery Box

Han Dynasty

Pottery

Mouth Diameter 17.8 cm/ Bottom Diameter 10 cm/ Height 10 cm/ Weight 750 g

子母口，无盖，直折腹，腹部上边有二道弦纹，
平底。完整无损。容器。陕西省西安市征集。

陕西医史博物馆藏

This box has a snap button without the lid, a
straight body, decorated with two string patterns,
tapering to a flat bottom. This well-preserved
vessel was collected from Xi'an, Shaanxi
Province.

Preserved in Shaanxi Museum of Medical History

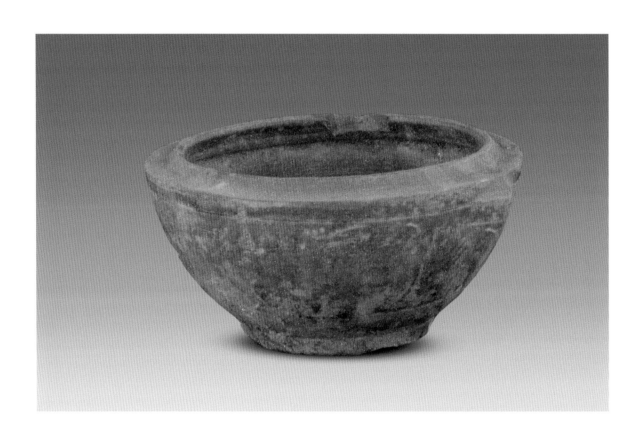

陶盒

汉

釉陶质

口径 14 厘米，底径 9 厘米，通高 9 厘米，重 800 克

Pottery Box

Han Dynasty

Glazed Pottery

Mouth Diameter 14 cm/ Bottom Diameter 9 cm/ Height 9 cm/ Weight 800 g

子母口，斜腹，圈足，腹部雕刻有花纹饰，
绿釉色。完整无损。容器。陕西省西安市长
安区康申利上交征集。

陕西医史博物馆藏

This box features a snap lid, and a body incised
with floral motifs tapering to a ring foot. This
green-glazed vessel remains intact, and was
donated by Kang Shenli in Chang'an District,
Xi'an City, Shaanxi Province.

Preserved in Shaanxi Museum of Medical History

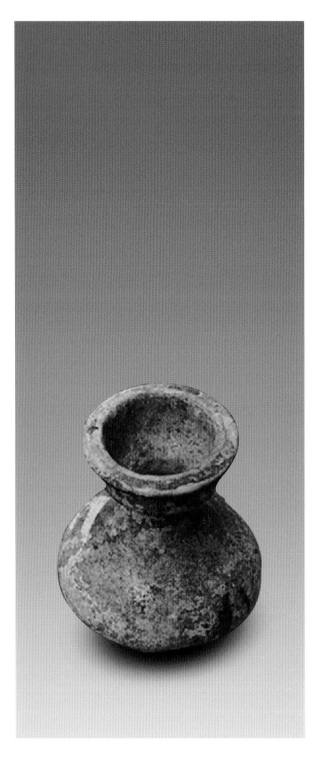

银釉唾壶

汉

陶质

上口直径 5.8 厘米，底部直径 7.8 厘米，壶身
直径 11.1 厘米，高 12.3 厘米

鼓腹，细短颈，敞口，侈唇外翻。卫生用具。

广东中医药博物馆藏

Silver-glazed Spittoon

Han Dynasty

Pottery

Upper Mouth Diameter 5.8 cm/ Bottom Diameter
7.8 cm/ Belly Diameter 11.1 cm/ Height 12.3 cm
The spittoon has a rounded belly, a short and
narrow neck and a wide flared mouth with an
everted rim. It was used as a sanitary appliance.
Preserved in Guangdong Chinese Medicine Museum

陶痰盂

汉

灰陶质

口径 19.8 厘米，底径 9.5 厘米，通高 21 厘米，重 1750 克

口呈大喇叭口形，鼓腹，平底，肩部有二道弦纹。稍残，口沿有修补。卫生器具。陕西省铜川市征集。

陕西医史博物馆藏

Pottery Spittoon

Han Dynasty

Grey Pottery

Mouth Diameter 19.8 cm/ Bottom Diameter 9.5 cm / Height 21 cm/ Weight 1,750 g

The spittoon has a large trumpet-shaped mouth, a globular belly, a flat bottom and a shoulder decorated with double rings of string patterns. The spittoon is slightly damaged and has its mouth rim restored. It was used as a sanitary appliance, and was collected from Tongchuan City, Shaanxi Province.

Preserved in Shaanxi Museum of Medical History

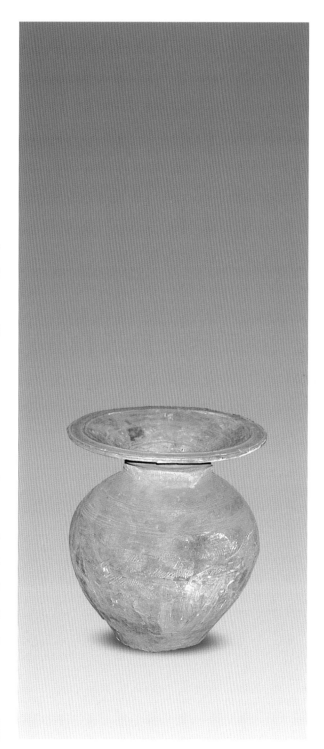

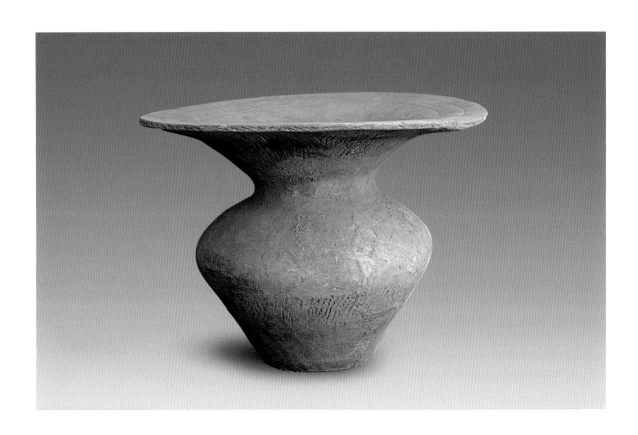

陶痰盂

汉

陶质

口径 28.5 厘米，底径 10 厘米，高 20.8 厘米，重 2300 克

Pottery Spittoon

Han Dynasty

Pottery

Mouth Diameter 28.5 cm/ Bottom Diameter 10 cm /Height 20.8 cm/ Weight 2,300 g

大喇叭，束颈，折腹，平底，口沿背部及下
腹部饰有绳纹。口沿有裂印。生活器具。陕
西省西安古玩市场征集。

陕西医史博物馆藏

The spittoon has a huge trumpet-shaped mouth,
a waisted neck, a tapering ovoid body and a
flat bottom. Under the back of the mouth rim
and around the lower belly are decorated with
rope patterns respectively. Crackles can be seen
on the mouth rim. It was used as a household
utensil for daily use, and was collected from
Xi'an Antiques Market, Shaanxi Province.
Preserved in Shaanxi Museum of Medical History

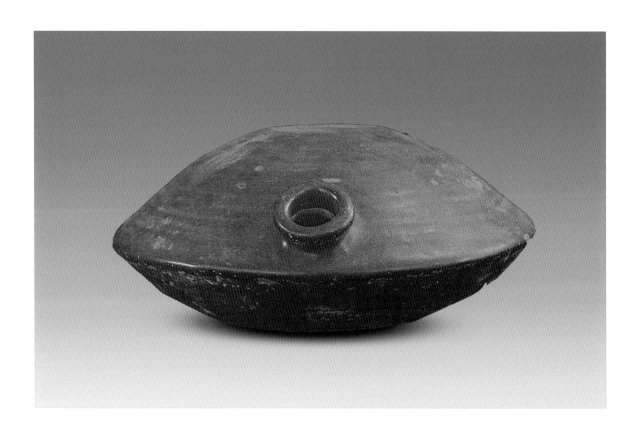

尿壶

汉

陶质

直径 28.5 厘米，通高 12 厘米，重 2650 克

Chamber Pot

Han Dynasty

Pottery

Diameter 28.5 cm/ Height 12 cm/ Weight 2,650 g

龟形，棕色。完整无损。溺器。陕西历史博

物馆调拨。

陕西医史博物馆藏

The brown urinal vessel, in the shape of a turtle,

remains intact. It was allocated from Shaanxi

History Museum.

Preserved in Shaanxi Museum of Medical History

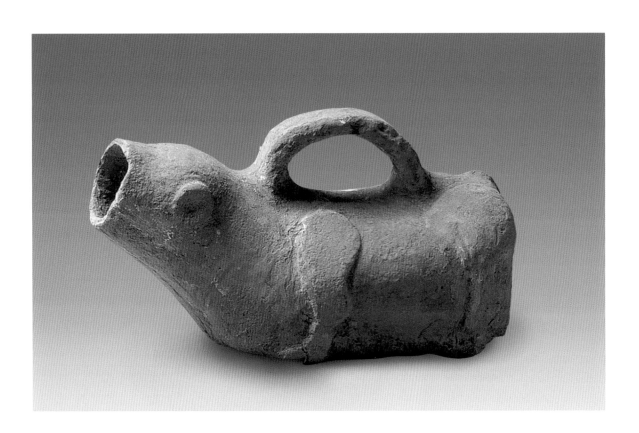

灰陶虎子

汉

灰陶质

长 26 厘米，宽 10 厘米，高 15.2 厘米

Grey Pottery "Huzi" (Tiger-shaped Chamber Pot)

Han Dynasty

Grey Pottery

Length 26 cm/ Width 10 cm/ Height 15.2 cm

虎昂首圆口，圆睁双目，四肢屈于腹两侧，背有弧形提梁。虎子是汉代到六朝墓葬中常见的随葬品，以其形似伏虎而得名。其为溺器，但也有学者认为是水器。南京市中央门外丘家山出土。

南京市博物馆藏

The chamber pot is in the shape of a tiger with its head up, its mouth and eyes wide open. It has four limbs crooked on both sides of the body and an arched loop handle on its back. The pot was named "Huzi" (tiger-shaped) due to its resemblance to a crouching tiger. It was a burial object commonly found in the tombs from the Han Dynasty to the Six Dynasties. It served as a urinal vessel, but some scholars hold that it should be a water container. The collection was unearthed at Qiujia Mountain outside of the Central Gate in Nanjing City, Jiangsu Province. Preserved in Nanjing Museum

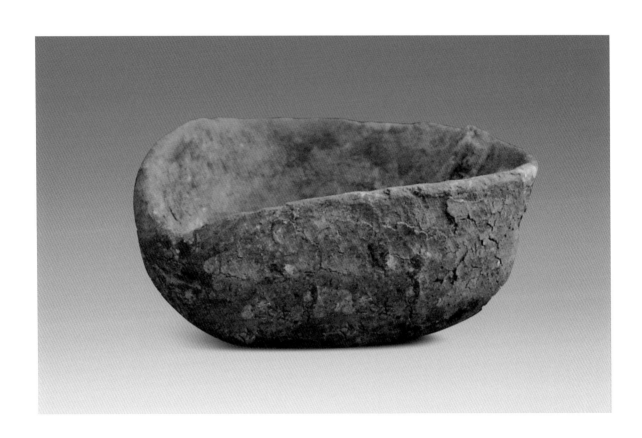

陶灯盏

汉

陶质

口径 10 厘米，底径 7 厘米，通高 4 厘米，重 200 克

Pottery Oil Lamp

Han Dynasty

Pottery

Mouth Diameter 10 cm/ Bottom Diameter 7 cm /Height 4 cm/ Weight 200 g

口为三角形状，有流口，平底，粗糙。完整
无损。生活用器具，照明灯具。

陕西医史博物馆藏

This roughly-made lamp has a triangle mouth
with an opening on its rim and a flat bottom.
Used for lighting, this daily household utensil
remains intact.

Preserved in Shaanxi Museum of Medical History

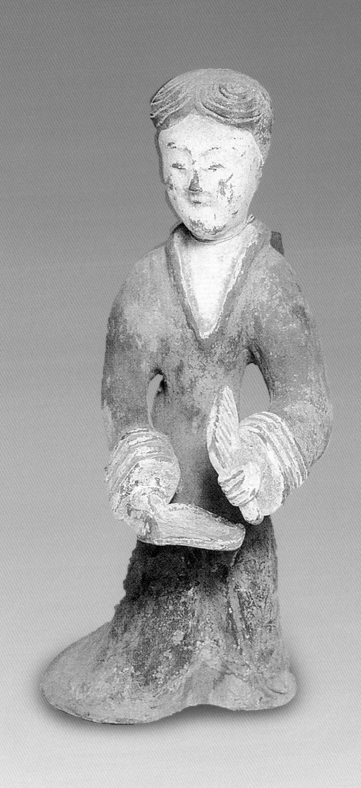

笤帚俑（明器）

汉

陶质

宽 13 厘米，高 28 厘米

此为女性俑，右手持一簸箕，左手握笤帚。

河南洛阳出土。

北京中医药大学中医药博物馆藏

Figurine Holding Broom (Burial Object)

Han Dynasty

Pottery

Width 13 cm/ Height 28 cm

This female figurine is holding a dustpan in her right hand and a broom in her left hand. It was unearthed in Luoyang City, Henan Province.

Preserved in the Museum of Chinese Medical, Beijing University of Chinese Medicine

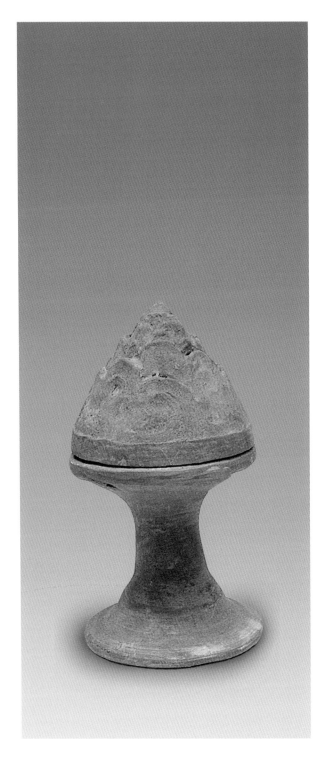

熏炉

汉

陶质

高 19.4 厘米

由灰陶制成，下部为高圈足形，上部为山形。
属于熏香用具。由洛阳市文物商店征集。

　　　　成都中医药大学中医药传统文化博物馆藏

Censer

Han Dynasty

Pottery

Height 19.4 cm

This grey pottery censer has a high ring foot and
a top designed in the shape of a mountain. The
censer was used as a household utensil for daily
use, and was collected from an antique shop in
Luoyang City, Henan Province.

Preserved in Museum of Traditional Chinese
Medicine Culture, Chengdu University of Traditional
Chinese Medicine

熏炉

汉

陶质

高 17.3 厘米

绿釉红陶，底部为盘形，器身作豆状，上有山
形盖，盖上有孔，便于香气溢出。由洛阳市文
物商店征集。

　　成都中医药大学中医药传统文化博物馆藏

Censer

Han Dynasty

Pottery

Height 17.3 cm

This red pottery censer, coated with green glaze,
has a plate-shaped bottom and a bean-shaped body.
There is a design of mountain on the porous lid
with holes, which can facilitate aroma diffusion.
The object was collected from an antique shop in
Luoyang City, Henan Province.

Preserved in Museum of Traditional Chinese
Medicine Culture, Chengdu University of Traditional
Chinese Medicine

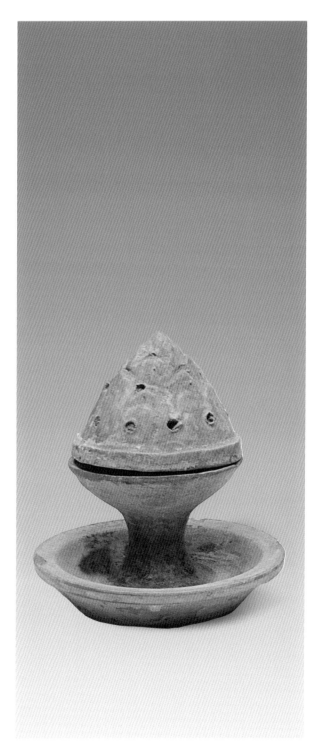

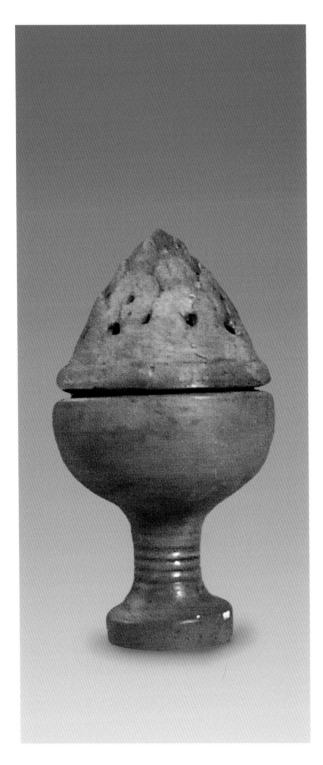

陶熏炉

汉

陶质

底径 7.2 厘米，腹径 12.2 厘米，通高 21.7 厘米

Pottery Censer

Han Dynasty

Pottery

Bottom Diameter 7.2 cm/ Belly Diameter 12.2 cm/

Height 21.7 cm

此熏炉也称"琉璃陶博山炉"。黄褐陶烧制。
棕黄色釉，下部呈高脚杯状，饰螺纹，上配
镂空花蕾尖状盖，造型美观。保存基本完好。
熏香用具。

中华医学会／上海中医药大学医史博物馆藏

This censer, also known as "Glazed Pottery
Censer with Boshan-style Design", is covered
with brown glaze. Its lower body is in the
shape of the high ring foot decorated with
spiral patterns, raising to a bud-shaped lid with
openwork. This elegantly shaped censer, used
as incense burner, has been kept in good shape.
Preserved in Chinese Medical Association/
Museum of Chinese Medicine, Shanghai
University of Traditional Chinese Medicine

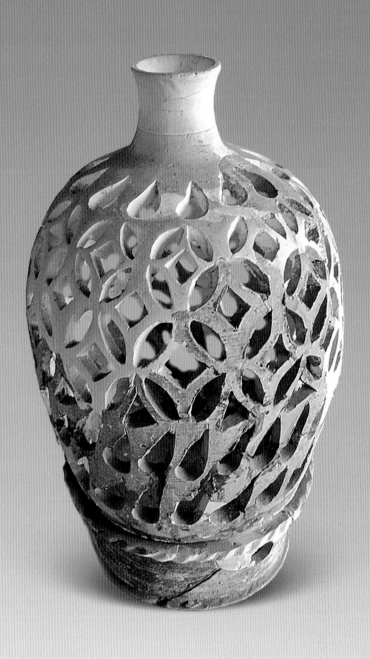

熏

汉

陶质

高 44 厘米

器身镂空，有底座。残损较严重。由成都市考

古队调拨。

　　成都中医药大学中医药传统文化博物馆藏

Censer

Han Dynasty

Pottery

Height 44 cm

The censer has a hollowed-out body and a base,

which is severely damaged. It was allocated from

Archaeological Team of Chengdu City.

Preserved in Museum of Traditional Chinese Medicine

Culture, Chengdu University of Traditional Chinese

Medicine

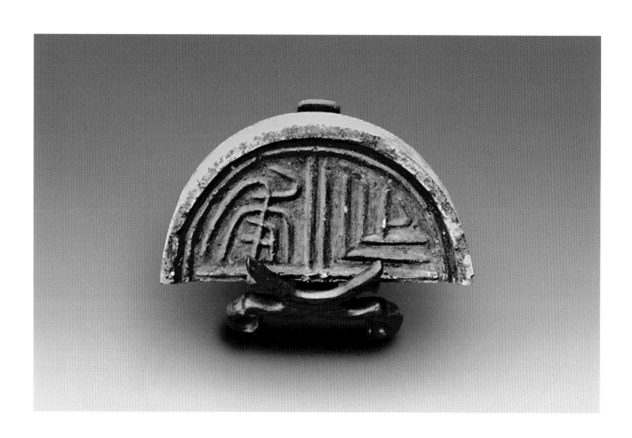

延年瓦当（带架）

汉

陶质

高 8.8 厘米，直径 16.8 厘米

Tile-end with Characters "Yan Nian"(With a Stand)

Han Dynasty

Pottery

Height 8.8 cm/ Diameter 16.8 cm

半圆形，上有"延年"二字，用于装饰。秦汉之后，盛行圆形。

广东中医药博物馆藏

The semicircle tile-end is decorated with two Chinese characters "Yan Nian" (longevity). The round tile-ends became prevailing after the Qin and Han dynasties.

Preserved in Guangdong Chinese Medicine Museum

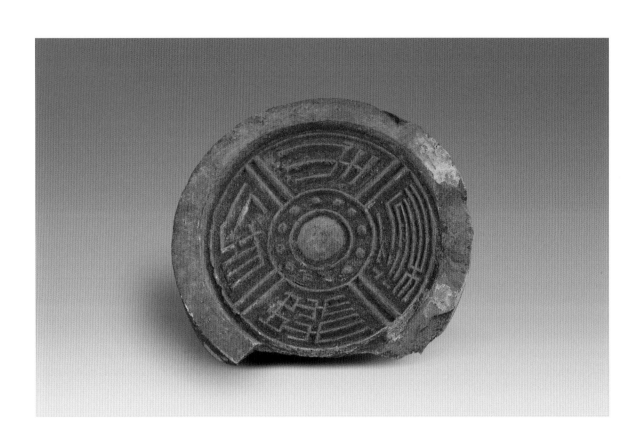

瓦当

汉

陶质

直径 17.6 厘米，通高 3.5 厘米，重 900 克

面上有字"万寿无疆"。有残。建筑构件。

陕西医史博物馆藏

Tile-end

Han Dynasty

Pottery

Diameter 17.6 cm/ Height 3.5 cm/ Weight 900 g

The tile-end is decorated with an inscription of four Chinese characters "Wan Shou Wu Jiang" (eternal life). The damaged piece was used as an architectural unit.

Preserved in Shaanxi Museum of Medical History

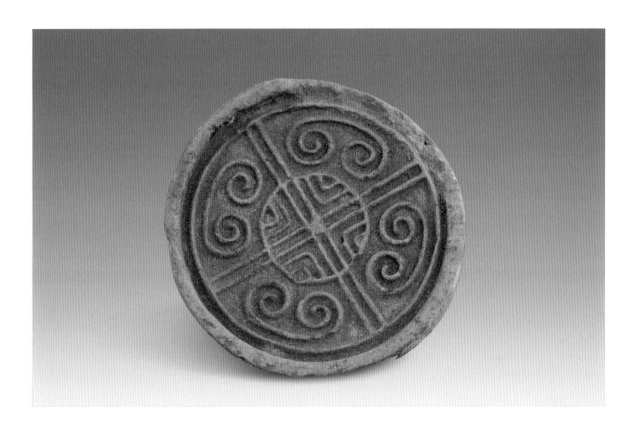

瓦当

汉

陶质

直径 14.5 厘米，通高 3 厘米，重 600 克

外沿上突，外周云纹，中间雷纹。有残。建筑构件。

陕西医史博物馆藏

Tile-end

Han Dynasty

Pottery

Diameter 14.5cm/ Height 3 cm/ Weight 600 g

With a convex outer rim, the tile-end is decorated with cloud patterns at the peripheral area and thunder patterns in the centre. The broken piece was used as an architectural unit.

Preserved in Shaanxi Museum of Medical History

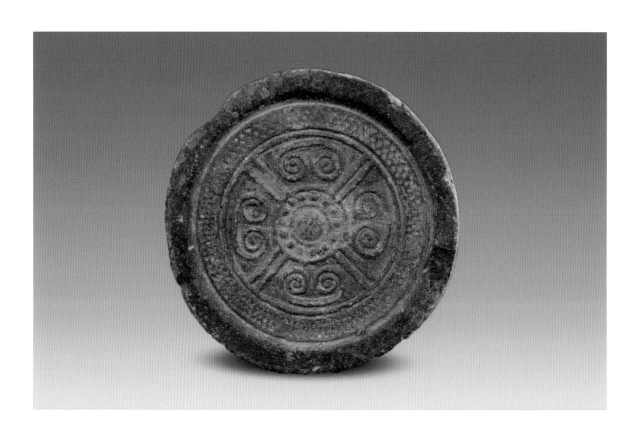

瓦当

汉

陶质

直径 15.5 厘米，通高 3 厘米，重 550 克

Tile-end

Han Dynasty

Pottery

Diameter 15.5 cm/ Height 3 cm /Weight 550 g

面上云纹，中间蔡花纹。有残。建筑构件。

陕西医史博物馆藏

The tile-end is decorated with cloud patterns on the surface and sunflower patterns in the centre. The broken piece was used as an architectural unit.

Preserved in Shaanxi Museum of Medical History

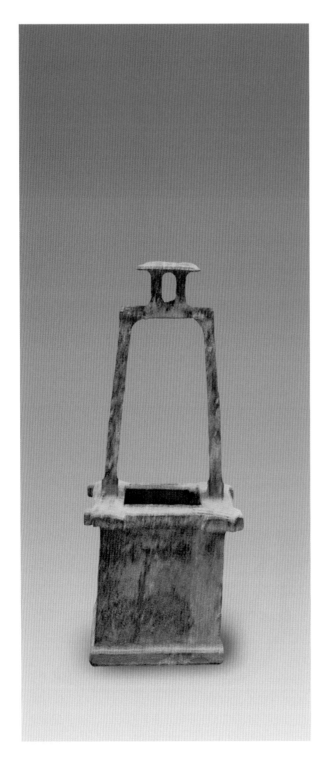

水井

汉

陶质

底为 11 厘米 × 11 厘米，高 30 厘米

施绿釉，有井架的造型。

成都中医药大学中医药传统文化博物馆藏

Well

Han Dynasty

Pottery

Bottom 11cm×11 cm/ Height 30 cm

The well is green glazed and modelled with a well curb.

Preserved in Museum of Traditional Chinese Medicine Culture, Chengdu University of Traditional Chinese Medicine

井

汉

陶质

井台16.5厘米×16.5厘米，底14厘米×14厘米，

高22厘米

属常见的汉代水井模型，有井台。部分已残。

由成都市考古队调拨。

　　　　成都中医药大学中医药传统文化博物馆藏

Well

Han Dynasty

Pottery

Length of Platform 16.5 cm×16.5 cm/ Width of

Platform 14 cm×14 cm/ Height 22 cm

It is a common well model with a platform in the

Han Dynasty. It was partly damaged. It was allocated

from Archaeological Team of Chengdu City.

Preserved in Museum of Traditional Chinese

Medicine Culture, Chengdu University of Traditional

Chinese Medicine

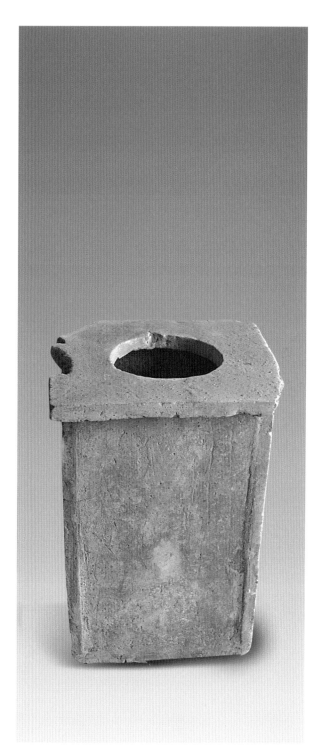

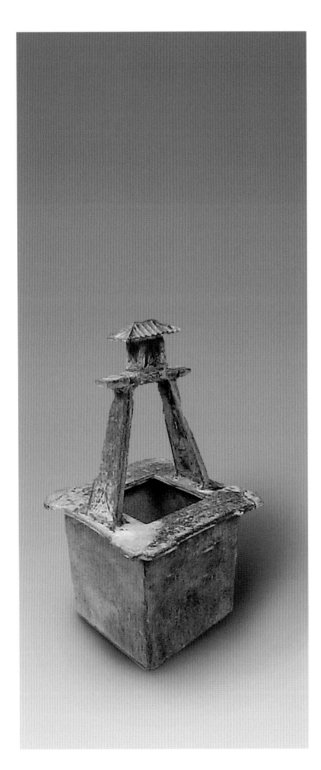

陶方井

汉

灰黑陶质

井沿 20.9 厘米 ×20.3 厘米，底 15.8×15.8 厘米，通高 36.5 厘米

Square Pottery Well

Han Dynasty

Greyish-black Pottery

Platform 20.9 cm×20.3 cm/ Bottom 15.8 cm×15.8 cm/

Height 36.5 cm

圆筒状，上部有井栏，栏上附有水桶一只，下部呈圆筒状，施青黄釉。基本保存完好。为明器。

中华医学会 / 上海中医药大学医史博物馆藏

This cylinder-shaped well has a bucket attached to the well curb on its upper body, and its lower body is circular in shape. It is covered with greenish-yellow glaze. This burial object is basically preserved in good condition.

Preserved in Chinese Medical Association/ Museum of Chinese Medicine, Shanghai University of Traditional Chinese Medicine

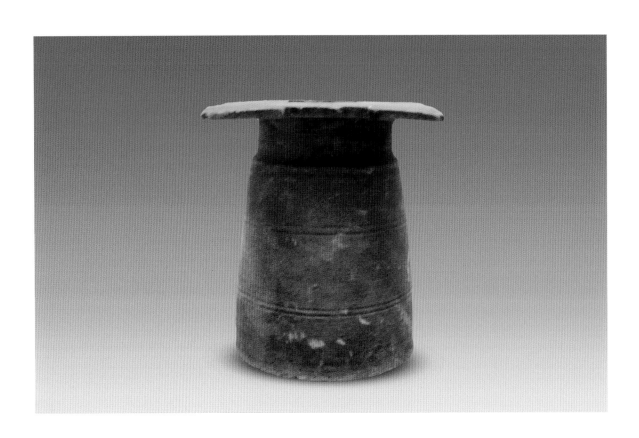

水井

汉

陶质

平台为 22 厘米 × 22 厘米，高 27 厘米

Well

Han Dynasty

Pottery

Platform 22 cm×22 cm/ Height 27 cm

井台为方形，井身上小下大。为当时水井的
模型。由成都市考古队调拨。

　　成都中医药大学中医药传统文化博物馆藏

With a square platform, the well has a gradually
spreading body, which is a model of the well
in the Han Dynasty. It was allocated from
Archaeological Team of Chengdu City.
Preserved in Museum of Traditional Chinese
Medicine Culture, Chengdu University of
Traditional Chinese Medicine

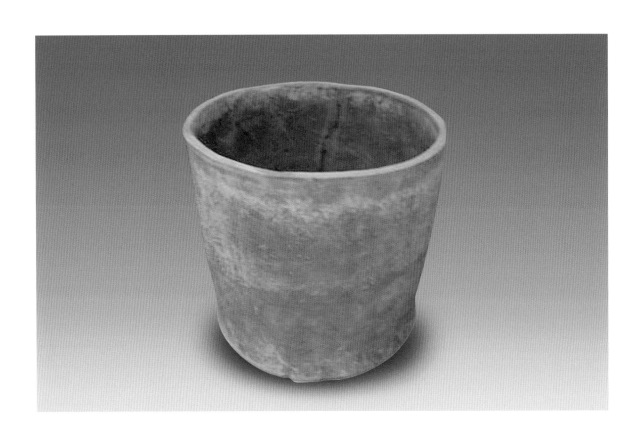

井圈

汉

陶质

口径 70 厘米，高 60 厘米

此为打井时所用的材料，在成都平原十分常见。
由成都市考古队调拨。

成都中医药大学中医药传统文化博物馆藏

Well Walling

Han Dynasty

Pottery

Mouth Diameter 7 cm/ Height 60 cm

This utensil was very commonly used for well digging in Chengdu Plain. It was allocated from Archaeological Team of Chengdu City.

Preserved in Museum of Traditional Chinese Medicine Culture, Chengdu University of Traditional Chinese Medicine

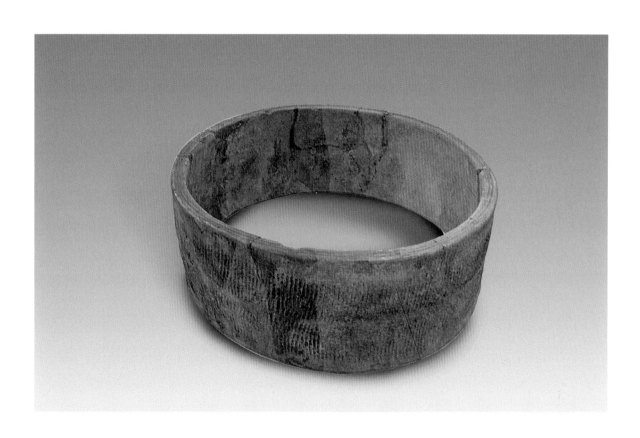

井圈

汉

陶质

高 18.5 厘米，口径 50 厘米

打井时所用的材料，在成都平原十分常见。由成都市考古队调拨。

成都中医药大学中医药传统文化博物馆藏

Well Walling

Han Dynasty

Pottery

Height 18.5 cm/ Mouth Diameter 50 cm

This utensil was very commonly used for well digging in Chengdu Plain. It was allocated from Archaeological Team of Chengdu City.

Preserved in Museum of Traditional Chinese Medicine Culture, Chengdu University of Traditional Chinese Medicine

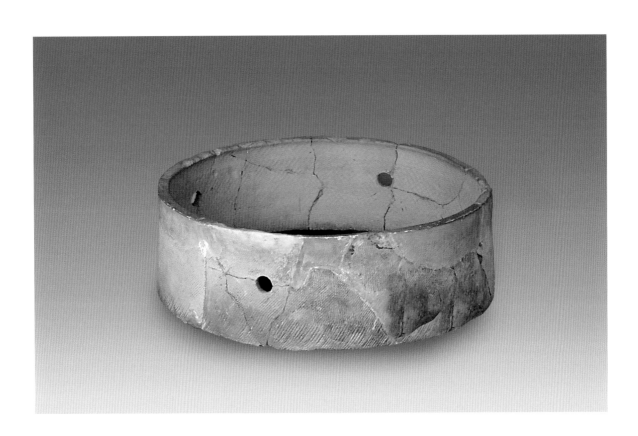

陶井圈

汉

陶质

直径 70 厘米，通高 24 厘米

Well Walling

Han Dynasty

Pottery

Diameter 71 cm/ Height 24 cm

此为水井建筑部件。该藏灰陶制成，圆筒形，表面有小孔，有修复痕迹。保存基本完好。

中华医学会 / 上海中医药大学医史博物馆藏

This cylindrical utensil is a part of a set of well construction. Though preserved basically in good shape, this grey pottery collection has small holes in the surface where restoration traces can be seen.

Preserved in Chinese Medical Association/ Museum of Chinese Medicine, Shanghai University of Traditional Chinese Medicine

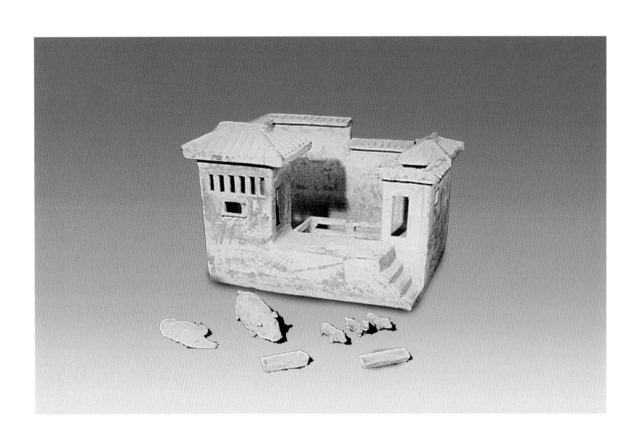

陶厕猪圈（明器）

汉

陶质

长 44 厘米，宽 35.5 厘米，高 31.5 厘米

Pottery Pigsty Connected with Toilet (Burial Object)

Han Dynasty

Pottery

Length 44 cm/ Width 35.5 cm/ Height 31.5 cm

四周围壁，两侧高台上筑厕所两间；高台下、围壁内为猪圈，内有母猪育仔及猪食槽模型。明器，反映了当时人对环境卫生的重视。

中国医史博物馆藏

This collection is surrounded by walls on four sides, and two toilets built on both sides of the high terrace. Under the terrace is the pigsty where the models of a sow with piglets nursing and the trough are located. The structure of this burial object shows that great emphasis was placed on environmental hygiene at that time.

Preserved in Chinese Medical History Museum

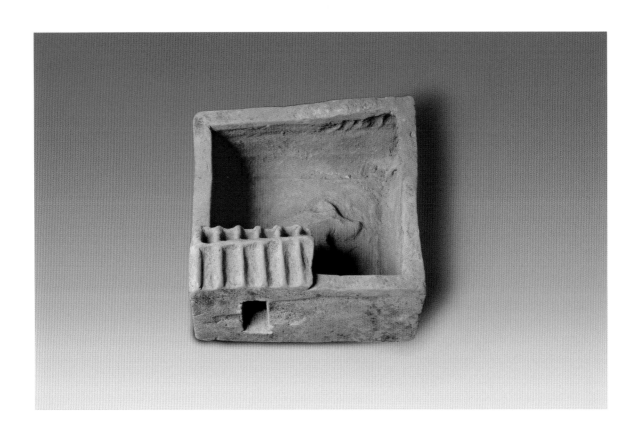

陶猪圈

汉

灰陶质

边长 16 厘米

Pottery Pigsty

Han Dynasty

Grey Pottery

Side Length 16 cm

平面略作方形，圈四周有墙，内卧一猪。一角塑房顶并开窗，反映汉代南京地区的家畜饲养状况。丧葬明器。南京出土。

南京市博物馆藏

With the plane nearly in square shape and a pig lying in it, the pigsty is surrounded by walls on four sides. On one of the corners is moulded the roof with a window, which reflects the cattle breeding conditions of the Han Dynasty in Nanjing region. This collection served as a burial object, and was unearthed in Nanjing City, Jiangsu Province.

Preserved in Nanjing Museum

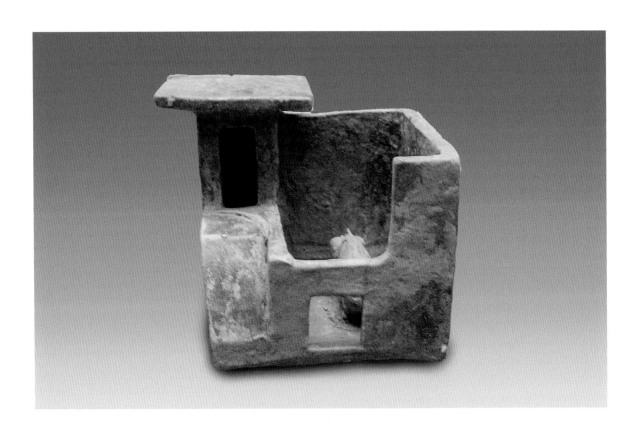

厕圈

汉

陶胎绿釉

长 22.2 厘米，宽 20.3 厘米，高 24 厘米

Toilet Connected with Pigsty

Han Dynasty

Green-glazed Pottery

Length 22.2 cm/ Width 20.3 cm/ Height 24 cm

方形，坡形通道，厕顶为平形，厕与圈相连，圈墙底有排气口和矩形清扫窗口，圈内有一陶胎绿釉猪模型，器形完整，制作精巧，为做工较为精致的明器，反映了墓葬主人对环境卫生的要求较高。洛阳出土，于 1999 年调拨至成都中医药大学中医药传统文化博物馆。

成都中医药大学中医药传统文化博物馆藏

This square collection has a ramp leading up towards the toilet with a flat roof. A vent hole and a rectangular window for cleaning can be seen on the bottom of the enclosure. Next to the toilet, the pigsty encloses the model of a green-glazed pottery pig. In good shape and with exquisite workmanship, this collection served as a burial object which shows the high requirement of the tomb owner for environmental hygiene conditions. Unearthed in Luoyang City, it was transferred to the Museum of Traditional Chinese Medical Culture, Chengdu University of Traditional Chinese Medicine in 1999.

Preserved in Museum of Traditional Chinese Medicine Culture, Chengdu University of Traditional Chinese Medicine

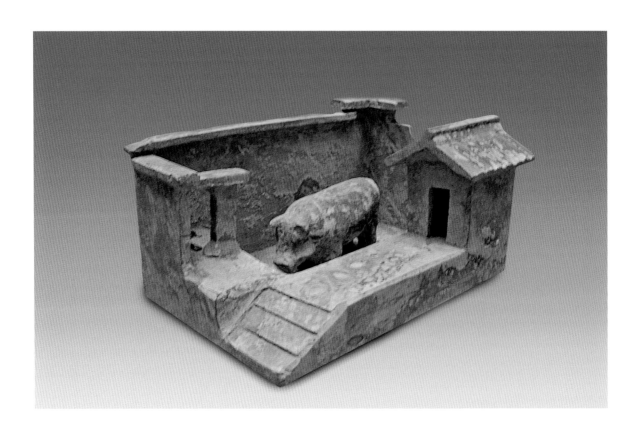

厕圈

汉

灰陶质

长 36.7 厘米，宽 26 厘米，高 17.7 厘米

Toilet Connected with Pigsty

Han Dynasty

Grey Pottery

Length 36.7 cm/ Width 26 cm/ Height 17.7 cm

长方形，台阶形通道，圈与厕相连，内有一灰陶猪模型，器形完好，为随葬用的明器。此器真实地反映了汉代厕所的情况：多将其建于猪圈之上，设有供上下的通道，正面有门，或设有气窗，室内地板中留有长方形孔洞，下通猪圈，此种形式在目前我国农村很多地方仍可见到，说明我国环境卫生意识由来已久。洛阳出土，于1999年调拨至成都中医药大学中医药传统文化博物馆。

成都中医药大学中医药传统文化博物馆藏

This rectangular collection has a ramp with steps leading up towards the toilet connected to the pigsty, which encloses a model of a grey pottery pig. This burial object, in good shape, shows the authentic conditions of the toilet in Han Dynasty. Often built above the pigsty, the toilet has a path to go up and down, a front door or a transom window, and a rectangular hole left on the indoor floor open to the pigsty. This kind of design is still in use in the countryside of China at present, a clear evidence that the awareness of environmental hygiene is long-standing in China. Unearthed in Luoyang City, this object was transferred to Preserved in Museum of Traditional Chinese Medicine Culture, Chengdu University of Traditional Chinese Medicine in 1999.

Preserved in Museum of Traditional Chinese Medicine Culture, Chengdu University of Traditional Chinese Medicine

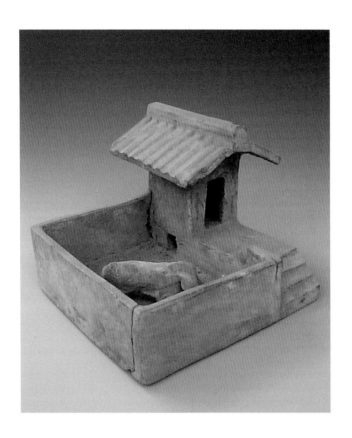

陶猪圈

汉

灰陶质

长 22 厘米，宽 19.8 厘米，高 16.3 厘米

Pottery Pigsty

Han Dynasty

Grey Pottery

Length 22 cm/ Width 19.8 cm/ Height 16.3 cm

猪圈状，猪圈和厕所连为一体，有台阶通往厕所，猪圈内有一陶猪，工艺粗糙。明器。保存基本完好。

中华医学会 / 上海中医药大学医史博物馆藏

The object is in the shape of a pigsty, connected to a toilet by steps. In the pigsty a pottery pig with rough workmanship can be seen. It served as a burial object and has been kept basically in good condition.

Preserved in Chinese Medical Association/ Museum of Chinese Medicine, Shanghai University of Traditional Chinese Medicine

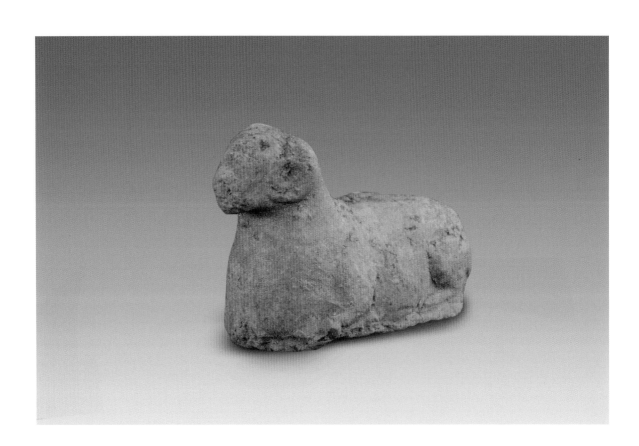

陶羊

汉

红陶质

长径 10 厘米，底径 9.5 厘米，通高 6.5 厘米，重 250 克

Pottery Sheep

Han Dynasty

Red Pottery

Long Diameter 10cm/ Bottom Diameter 9.5cm/ Height 6.5cm/ Weight 250g

陶羊呈卧状，双耳卷曲。陶塑，完整无损。
陕西省西安市长安区征集。

陕西医史博物馆收藏

The sheep is lying down with curly ears. It is intact and undamaged. It was collected from Chang'an District of Xi'an of Shaanxi province. Preserved in Shaanxi Medical History Museum

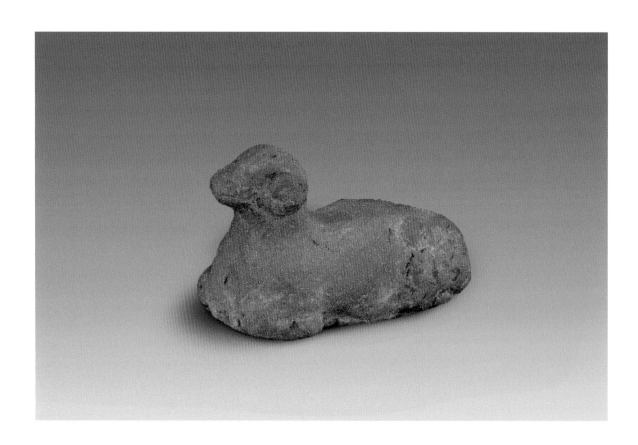

陶羊

汉

红陶质

通长径 10 厘米，通宽 5 厘米，高 6 厘米，2000 克

Pottery Sheep

Han Dynasty

Red Pottery

Long Diameter 10 cm/ Width 5 cm/ Height 6cm/ Weight 2,000g

卧羊状态。完整无损。明器，艺术品。陕西省西安市长安区康申利上交征集。

陕西医史博物馆收藏

The sheep is crouching on the ground. It is intact and undamaged. It is a funerary and art ware. It was collected from Kang Shenli of Chang'an District of Xi'an City, Shaanxi province. Preserved in Shaanxi Medical History Museum

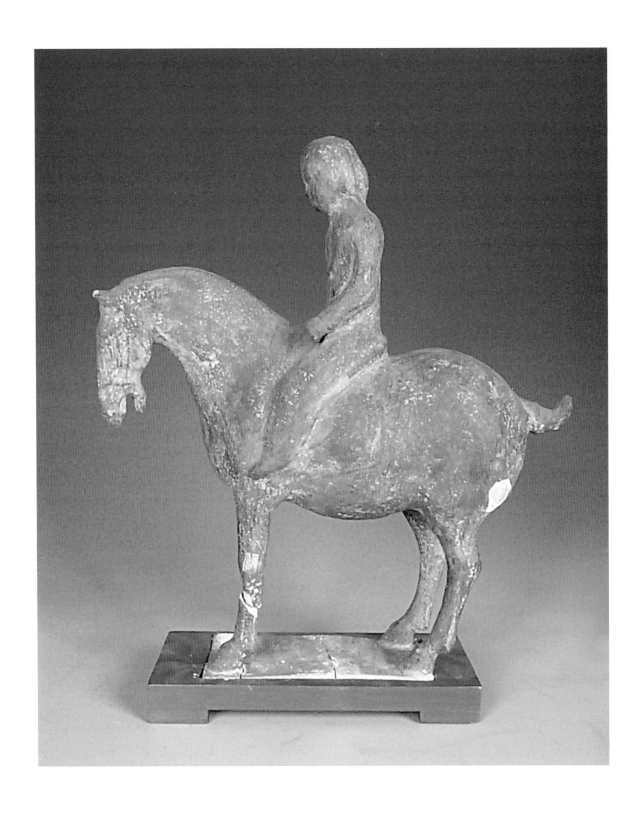

骑士俑

汉

陶质

通长 34.4 厘米，通高 38.8 厘米

该藏为黑灰色，马身肥硕，四肢直立，马尾
短小上扬，背上骑有人俑，造型美观。两前
马腿均断开。人骑马形。明器。1955 年入藏。

　中华医学会 / 上海中医药大学医史博物馆藏

Figurine of a Knight

Pottery

Han Dynasty

Length 34.4 cm/ Height 38.8 cm

It is beautifully shaped. The big and fleshy
horse is standing upright with its short tail
rising upward. A man is riding on the back of
the horse. Unfortunately, its front legs are both
broken. The dark gray horse riding figurine is
a funeral object. The figurine was collected in
the year of 1955.

Preserved in Chinese Medical Association/
Museum of Chinese Medicine, Shanghai
University of Traditional Chinese Medicine

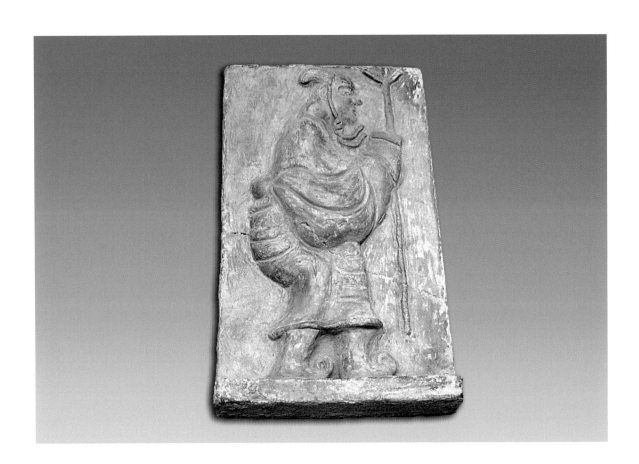

画像砖

汉

陶质

宽 17 厘米，高 27.5 厘米，厚 2 厘米

Portrait Brick

Han Dynasty

Width 17 cm/ Height 27.5 cm/ Thickness 2 cm

该画像砖为高浮雕的执仗俑图案，由学校教师捐赠。

　　成都中医药大学中医药传统文化博物馆藏

The brick portrait is the high-relief of a guard of honor. It was donated by a teacher.

Preserved in Museum of Traditional Chinese Medicine Culture, Chengdu University of Traditional Chinese Medicine

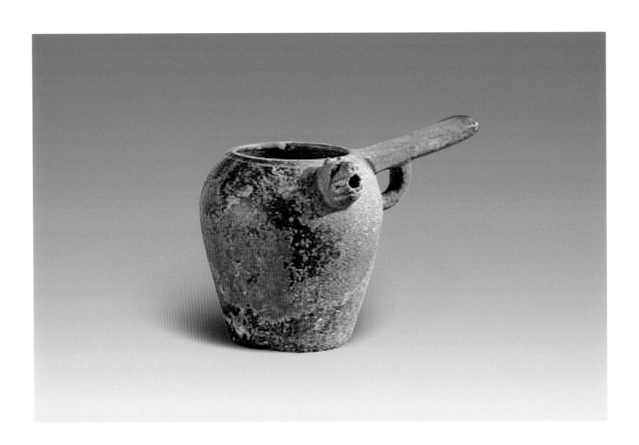

煎药锅

汉

黑陶质

腹径 18 厘米，底径 16 厘米，柄长 26 厘米，高 22 厘米

Medicine-boiling Pot

Han Dynasty

Black Pottery

Belly Diameter 18 cm/ Bottom Diameter 16 cm/ Length of Handle 26 cm/ Height 22 cm

敛口，溜肩，肩部塑有虎头型嘴和长执柄，柄根底部与桥形耳相连，斜腹，平底。煎药工具。

北京御生堂中医药博物馆藏

The pot has a contracted mouth, an inclined shoulder, a flat bottom and a narrow and inclined shoulder which is casted with long handle and the spout in the shape of a tiger's head. The end part of handle and bridge-shaped ear serves to connect and support. It was utilized for boiling medicine.

Preserved in Chinese Medicine Museum of Beijing Yu Sheng Tang Drugstore

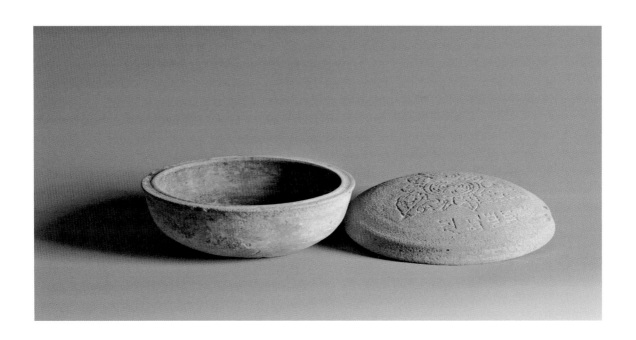

"吉祥"纹药盒

汉

陶质

腹径 12 厘米，高 10 厘米

Medicine Box with"Ji Xiang"Pattern

Han Dynasty

Pottery

Belly Diameter 12 cm/ Height 10 cm

子母口，直腹，圆底，平足，有盖，盖上刻花纹和文字，据考为"吉祥"之意。古时装药器皿。

北京御生堂中医药博物馆藏

The box has a cluster mouth, a vertical belly, a round base, flat feet and a lid with the flower patterns and characters which implies something propitious. It was used for medicine storage.

Preserved in Chinese Medicine Museum of Beijing Yu Sheng Tang Drugstore

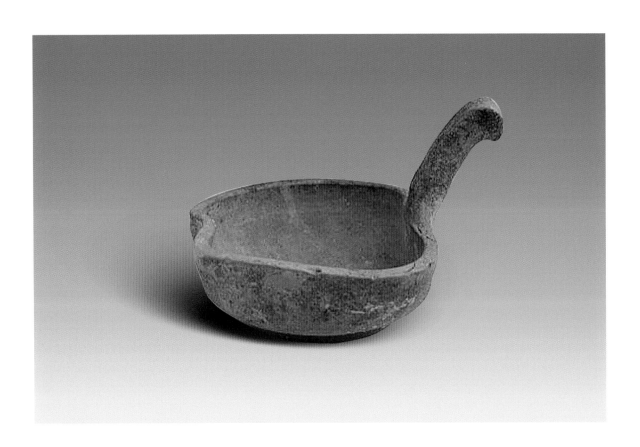

苹果型药勺

汉

陶质

口径 12 厘米，深 9 厘米，柄长 8 厘米

Apple-shaped Medicine Spoon

Han Dynasty

Pottery

Mouth Diameter 12 cm/ Depth 9 cm/ Handle Length 8 cm

苹果型，平沿，带把。古时熬药器具。

北京御生堂中医药博物馆藏

The spoon is shaped like an apple and has a flat edge with a handle. It was used as a tool for preparing medicine.

Preserved in Chinese Medicine Museum of Beijing Yu Sheng Tang Drugstore

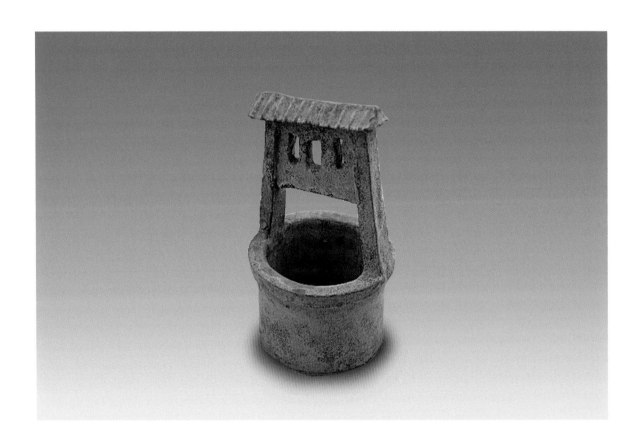

水井模型

汉

陶质

底径 18 厘米，高 26 厘米

Well Model

Han Dynasty

Pottery

Bottom Diameter 18 cm/ Height 26 cm

圆筒形井台，平沿，结水井沿上立亭蓬。亭蓬上塑有蓬顶，屋脊形上有瓦楞纹，两方形蓬柱与亭蓬间有梯形联，上有三个长方形孔错落相间，用于系栓掉水桶之井绳。亭蓬可防止脏东西进入水井。其与水井间有井台相隔，离地面有一段距离，亦可阻止脏水流入，防止脏东西进入，表明当时人已经很注意饮水卫生了。

北京御生堂中医药博物馆藏

The model has a cylindrical well stage, a flat rim with pavilion which was used for preventing the rubbish into the well. There is a roof on the top of pavilion and the corrugated patterns on the roof. Double square pillars and pavilion serve to connect in the shape of trapezoid, and there are three rectangle holes which were designed for hitching the well rope. The distance between pavilion and underground exists for the sake of preventing the wasted water and something dirty into it, which implies people in Han Dynasty cared about personal hygiene.

Preserved in Chinese Medicine Museum of Beijing Yu Sheng Tang Drugstore

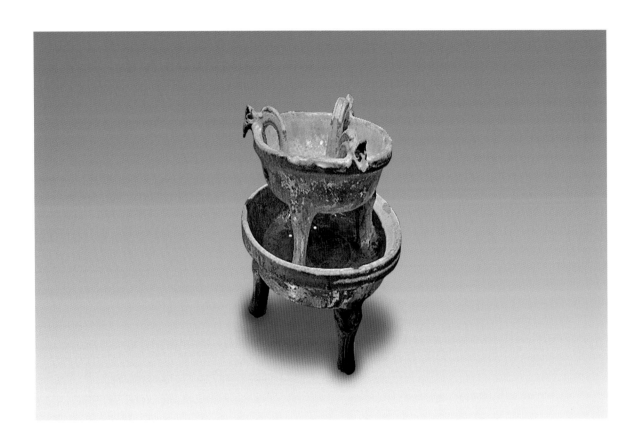

绿釉过滤器

汉

陶质

过滤直径 20 厘米，高 20 厘米

Green-glazed Filter

Han Dynasty

Pottery

Filter Diameter 20 cm/ Height 20 cm

红陶质，外施绿釉，分上下两部分，上为滤器，下为盛器，用于过滤中药残渣。上部敞口，三龙头伏于沿上，张口翘望，三桥形龙身探入器中，弧形底上有滤孔，三足玉龙首错落相隔。下部鼎形盛器，敞口，三足。

北京御生堂中医药博物馆藏

The exterior of red pottery filter is painted with green glaze. It is divided into two parts. The upper part is the filter which has a flared mouth. Three mouth-opened and cocking-up dragons' heads are lying on the rim. While three bridge-shaped parts stretched into the tool and the head of dragon with three feet is carved on the curved bottom with five holes. The lower part is the Ding vessel-shaped container which has a flared mouth and three feet, and was used for filtering the medicine.
Preserved in Chinese Medicine Museum of Beijing Yu Sheng Tang Drugstore

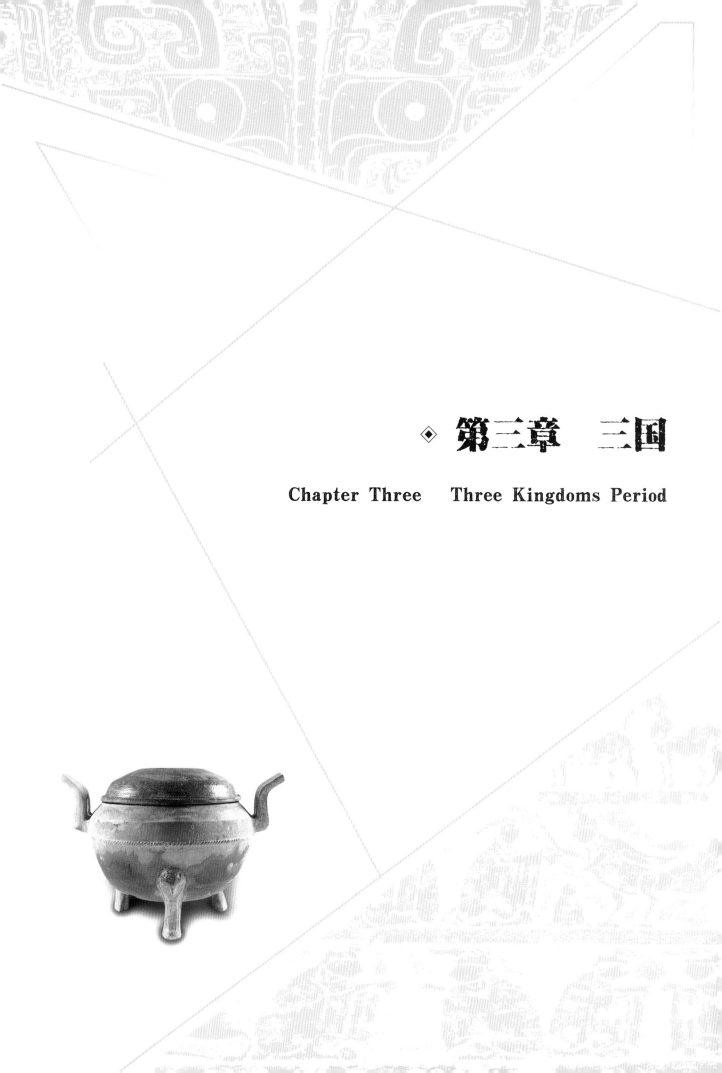

◆ 第三章 三国

Chapter Three　　Three Kingdoms Period

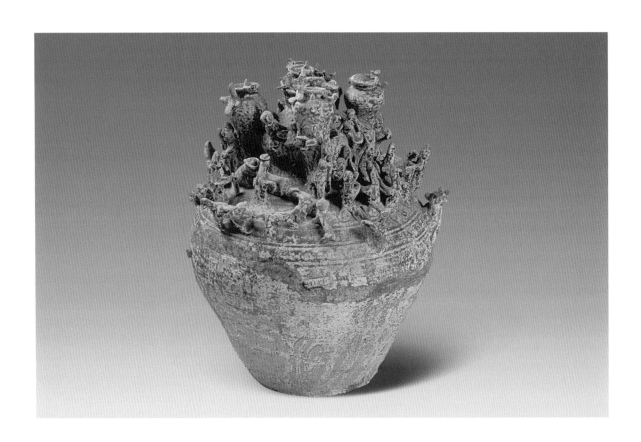

"孝子送葬" 褐釉陶魂瓶

三国·吴

釉陶质

口径 6.7 厘米，底径 15.5 厘米，高 36.7 厘米

Brown-glazed Pottery Soul Jar with Funeral Procession Design

Wu State of Three Kingdoms Period

Glazed Pottery

Mouth Diameter 6.7 cm/ Bottom Diameter 15.5 cm/ Height 36.7 cm

上部为一束颈圆肩的小罐，肩部附堆四个小罐；下部为一鼓腹平底罐。上部小罐尤其是罐口挤满了引颈振翅的雀鸟。下部的大罐上装饰繁缛，塑有人像二十一个，其中四人跪在棺木前，头缠孝巾；另一些为鼓瑟，鸣竽、吹笙、敲鼓的奏乐使人，似在为棺木中人送葬。其外还贴塑了狗、羊、兔、鸡等物。施褐釉，大罐腹部以下无釉。南京锅厂出土。

南京市博物馆藏

On the upper part of this soul jar is a small jar with a contracted neck and a rounded shoulder, on which four small jars are pasted, while the lower part is a big jar featuring a bulging profile and a flat bottom. There are birds swarming around the mouth of the smaller jars, with their necks stretching and wings flapping. Over-elaborate decorations can be seen on the lower bigger jar, on which twenty-one human figurines are modelled. Four of them are kneeling down in front of the coffin, with mourning towel twining around their forehead; the others are musicians playing Se (a type of standing harp with 5-25 strings), Yu (free reed mouth organ), Sheng (reed-pipe wind instrument) and Gu (drum), as if mourning for the departed person in the coffin. Appliqué animals like dogs, goats, rabbits and roosters are also modelled on the bigger jar. The soul jar is coated with brown glaze except the part under the abdomen. It was unearthed in a pot plant of Nanjing City, Jiangsu Province.

Preserved in Nanjing Museum

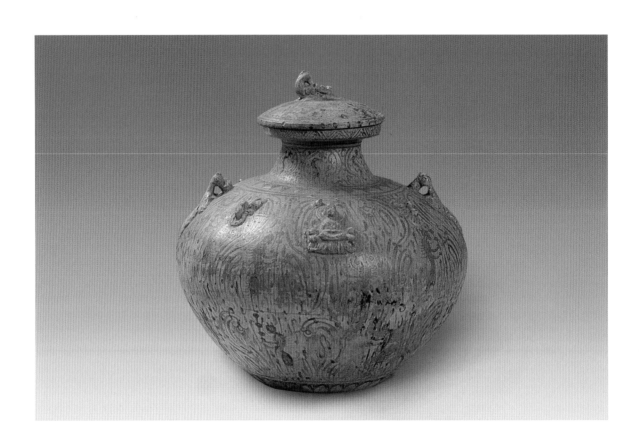

青釉羽人纹瓷盘口壶

三国·吴

瓷质

口径 12.6 厘米，底径 13.6 厘米，通高 32.1 厘米

Celadon Pot with a Dish-shaped Mouth and Design of Immortal Figures Holding Sceptre

Wu State of Three Kingdoms Period

Porcelain

Mouth Diameter 12.6 cm/ Bottom Diameter 13.6 cm/ Height 32.1 cm

盘口，短颈，圆鼓腹，有系，平底。盖贴塑一回首鸟为钮，周围绘两蒂纹及四组人首、鸟、仙草纹图案；盖内壁及盘口内外穿插仙草、云气、连弧、弦纹等。颈部绘七只异兽。肩部贴塑两尊佛像、四个铺首、两个双首连体鸟，三者相间排列，整齐有序。佛像螺髻，后有背光，跌坐于双狮莲花座上，双首连体鸟，尾作菩提叶状。器身贴塑的纹橡皆以褐彩勾勒。器腹绘二十一个持节羽人，分列上下两排，错落有致，两两相对，其间插绘飘忽欲动的仙草和云气纹。胫部绘一周仰莲纹。米黄色胎，通体施釉，釉呈青黄色。

南京市博物馆藏

The pot has a dish-shaped mouth, a short neck, a globular body, a flat bottom and rings. A bird looking back is moulded as the knob on the top of its lid. Around the bird are double-pedicle patterns and four sets of human heads, birds and mesona chinensis. The interior wall of the lid and the dish-shaped mouth are decorated with patterns of mesona chinensis, clouds, continuous arcs and strings. Seven rare beasts are painted around the neck of the pot. Two statues of Buddha alternate with four beast heads as well as two conjoined double-headed birds on the shoulder of the pot in good order. With spiral coil hair and backlights, Buddhas sit cross-legged on lotus seats decorated with two lions. The tail of the conjoined double-headed bird is in the shape of a Tilia Europaea. Brown rafter patterns are drawn on the body of the pot. Twenty-one immortal figures holding sceptres are painted on the belly of the pot in two rows, facing each other. Among them, vivid mesona patterns and cloud patterns can be seen. The shin of the pot is embellished with one circle of upturned lotus patterns. The pot has a creamy-coloured body coated with bluish-yellow glaze.

Preserved in Nanjing Museum

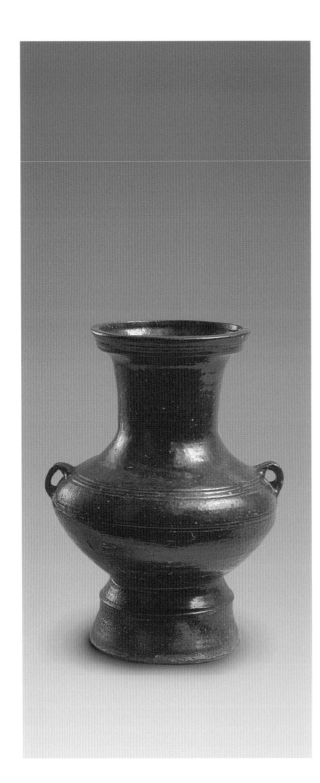

酱釉瓷钟

三国·吴

瓷质

口径 14.6 厘米，底径 14 厘米，高 28.6 厘米

Brown-glazed Pot

Wu State of Three Kingdoms Period

Porcelain

Mouth Diameter 14.6 cm/ Bottom Diameter 14 cm/

Height 28.6 cm

盘口外撇，直颈内收，肩至腹部呈鱼篓形，下承高圈足。肩部饰凹弦纹三周，其上置对称的竖形泥条状系。通体施酱黑釉，釉色明亮，造型规整。

南京市王谢古居陈列馆藏

This pot has a flared mouth in the shape of a plate and, a straight waisted neck. The part from the shoulder to the belly is in the shape of a fish basket, raised on a high ring foot. The shoulder is decorated with three concave rings, above which are two symmetrical rings in the form of a vertical clay bar. The whole body of the neatly-shaped pot is coated with lustrous brown glaze. Preserved in the Exhibition Hall in Wang Xie's Ancient Residence in Nanjing City

索 引

（馆藏地按拼音字母排序）

Index

Shanghai Museum of Traditional Chinese Medicine

参考文献

[1] 李经纬 . 中国古代医史图录 [M]. 北京：人民卫生出版社，1992.

[2] 傅维康，李经纬，林昭庚 . 中国医学通史：文物图谱卷 [M]. 北京：人民卫生出版社，2000.

[3] 和中浚，吴鸿洲 . 中华医学文物图集 [M]. 成都：四川人民出版社，2001.

[4] 上海中医药博物馆 . 上海中医药博物馆馆藏珍品 [M]. 上海：上海科学技术出版社，2013.

[5] 西藏自治区博物馆 . 西藏博物馆 [M]. 北京：五洲传播出版社，2005.

[6] 崔乐泉 . 中国古代体育文物图录：中英文本 [M]. 北京：中华书局，2000.

[7] 张金明，陆雪春 . 中国古铜镜鉴赏图录 [M]. 北京：中国民族摄影艺术出版社，2002.

[8] 文物精华编辑委员会 . 文物精华 [M]. 北京：文物出版社，1964.

[9] 谭维四 . 湖北出土文物精华 [M]. 武汉：湖北教育出版社，2001.

[10] 常州市博物馆 . 常州文物精华 [M]. 北京：文物出版社，1998.

[11] 镇江博物馆 . 镇江文物精华 [M]. 合肥：黄山书社，1997.

[12] 贵州省文化厅，贵州省博物馆 . 贵州文物精华 [M]. 贵阳：贵州人民出版社，2005.

[13] 徐良玉 . 扬州馆藏文物精华 [M]. 南京：江苏古籍出版社，2001.

[14] 昭陵博物馆，陕西历史博物馆 . 昭陵文物精华 [M]. 西安：陕西人民美术出版社，1991.

[15] 南通博物苑 . 南通博物苑文物精华 [M]. 北京：文物出版社，2005.

[16] 邯郸市文物研究所 . 邯郸文物精华 [M]. 北京：文物出版社，2005.

[17] 张秀生，刘友恒，聂连顺，等 . 中国河北正定文物精华 [M]. 北京：文化艺术出版社，1998.

[18] 陕西省咸阳市文物局 . 咸阳文物精华 [M]. 北京：文物出版社，2002.

[19] 安阳市文物管理局 . 安阳文物精华 [M]. 北京：文物出版社，2004.

[20] 深圳市博物馆 . 深圳市博物馆文物精华 [M]. 北京：文物出版社，1998.

[21]《中国文物精华》编辑委员会 . 中国文物精华（1993）[M]. 北京：文物出版社，1993.

[22] 夏路，刘永生 . 山西省博物馆馆藏文物精华 [M]. 太原：山西人民出版社，1999.

[23] 文物精华编辑委员会 . 文物精华 [M]. 北京：文物出版社，1957.

[24] 山西博物院，湖北省博物馆 . 荆楚长歌：九连墩楚墓出土文物精华 [M]. 太原：山西人民出版社，2011.

[25] 刘广堂，石金鸣，宋建忠 . 晋国雄风：山西出土两周文物精华 [M]. 沈阳：万卷出版公司，2009.

[26] 沈君山，王国平，单迎红 . 滦平博物馆馆藏文物精华 [M]. 北京：中国文联出版社，2012.

[27] 张家口市博物馆 . 张家口市博物馆馆藏文物精华 [M]. 北京：科学出版社，2011.

[28] 浙江省文物考古研究所 . 浙江考古精华 [M]. 北京：文物出版社，1999.

[29] 故宫博物院 . 故宫雕刻珍萃 [M]. 北京：紫禁城出版社，2004.

[30] 故宫博物院紫禁城出版社 . 故宫博物院藏宝录 [M]. 上海：上海文艺出版社，1986.

[31] 首都博物馆 . 大元三都 [M]. 北京：科学出版社，2016.

[32] 新疆维吾尔自治区博物馆 . 新疆出土文物 [M]. 北京：文物出版社，1975.

[33] 王兴伊，段逸山 . 新疆出土涉医文书辑校 [M]. 上海：上海科学技术出版社，2016.

[34] 刘学春 . 刍议医药卫生文物的概念与分类标准 [J]. 中华中医药杂志，2016，31（11）:4406-4409.

[35] 上海古籍出版社 . 中国艺海 [M]. 上海：上海古籍出版社，1994.

[36] 紫都，岳鑫 . 一生必知的 200 件国宝 [M]. 呼和浩特：远方出版社，2005.

[37] 谭维四 . 湖北出土文物精华 [M]. 武汉：湖北教育出版社，2001.

[38] 张建青 . 青海彩陶收藏与鉴赏 [M]. 北京：中国文史出版社，2007.

[39] 银景琦 . 仡佬族文物 [M]. 南宁：广西人民出版社，2014.

[40] 廖果，梁峻，李经纬 . 东西方医学的反思与前瞻 [M]. 北京：中医古籍出版社，2002.

[41] 梁峻，张志斌，廖果，等 . 中华医药文明史集论 [M]. 北京：中医古籍出版社，2003.

[42] 郑蓉，庄乾竹，刘聪，等 . 中国医药文化遗产考论 [M]. 北京：中医古籍出版社，2005.